100 Questions & Answers About Ovarian Cancer

THIRD EDITION

Don S. Dizon, MD, FACP

Clinical Co–Director, Gynecologic Oncology
Director, The Oncology Sexual Health Clinic
The Massachusetts General Hospital Cancer Center
Department of Medicine
Harvard Medical School
Boston, MA

Dorinda "Dee" Sparacio

CONTRIBUTORS

Nadeem R. Abu-Rustum, MD

Chief of the Gynecology Service,
Vice Chair for Technology Development, Department of Surgery,
Memorial Sloan Kettering Cancer Center, New York, NY

JONES & BARTLETT
LEARNING

World Headquarters
Jones & Bartlett Learning
5 Wall Street
Burlington, MA 01803
978-443-5000
info@jblearning.com
www.jblearning.com

Jones & Bartlett Learning books and products are available through most bookstores and online booksellers. To contact Jones & Bartlett Learning directly, call 800-832-0034, fax 978-443-8000, or visit our website, www.jblearning.com.

Production Credits

VP, Executive Publisher: David D. Cella
Executive Acquisitions Editor: Nancy Anastasi Duffy
Editorial Assistant: Jade Freeman
Associate Production Editor: Alex Schab
Digital Marketing Manager: Jennifer Sharp
Manufacturing and Inventory Control Supervisor: Amy Bacus
Composition: Miranda Design Studio, Inc.
Cover Design: Kristin E. Parker
Rights and Media Research Coordinator: Ashley Dos Santos
Cover Image: Top left: © iStockphoto/Thinkstock; Bottom left: © imagesource/123RF; Right: © Thinkstock
Printing and Binding: Edwards Brothers Malloy
Cover Printing: Edwards Brothers Malloy

Library of Congress Cataloging-in-Publication Data

Dizon, Don S.
  100 questions and answers about ovarian cancer / Don S. Dizon. — Third edition.
    pages cm
  ISBN 978-1-284-09028-4
  1. Ovaries—Cancer—Popular works. I. Title. II. Title: One hundred questions and answers about ovarian cancer.
  RC280.O8D55 2016
  616.99'465—dc23
                          2015006758

6048

Printed in the United States of America
19 18 17 16 15   10 9 8 7 6 5 4 3 2 1

DEDICATION

The third edition of this book is dedicated to the women I have had the pleasure and distinct honor to meet, to care for, and to partner with. It is in memory of those who have passed, especially the prior contributors, Andrea G. Brown, Zoe Ann King, Phyllis Hames, and Marsha Posusney, and to those who continue to live with ovarian cancer. It is further dedicated to my colleague, prior editor, and friend, Christopher B. Davis.

—Don S. Dizon, MD, FACP

CONTENTS

Introduction

In 2005, shortly after I was diagnosed with Stage 3B ovarian cancer, I searched online for books about ovarian cancer. One book, *100 Questions & Answers about Ovarian Cancer*, was written for patients, so I ordered a copy. As I read the first few sections of the book, I underlined and highlighted sections on staging, treatment, and side effect management. I also wrote notes to summarize the tips provided by Andrea Gibbs Brown, the book's coauthor who was an ovarian cancer survivor. When treatment ended, I put the book back on my bookshelf, thinking and hoping I would be in the small percentage of women who would never get a recurrence.

That was not the case, though. Two and a half years later, a CT scan showed disease on my spleen and liver. So I pulled the book off the shelf and started to read and highlight the parts of the book on Relapse (**Part Six**) and If Treatment Fails (**Part Seven**). I dog-eared the pages listing chemotherapy drugs and reread the section on side effect management. And I read, "Surgery for recurrent ovarian cancer is generally reserved for women whose disease recurs more than a year after completion ... whose tumors appear to the surgeon to be completely resectable (removable)." My tumors were resectable, and that is the option I chose in 2008.

When Dr. Don Dizon reached out to me to write the patient comments for the third edition of *100 Questions & Answers about Ovarian Cancer*, I walked over to my bookshelf and paged through the book. Then I wrote back and agreed to write the comments. I write these comments with the hope that I will be able to offer women and their caregivers the same support that the book's contents and Andrea's comments offered me 10 years ago.

As I started answering the questions, I was brought back to how I felt when my journey began. Ovarian cancer was not on my radar in 2005. The Consensus Statement on Ovarian Cancer Symptoms had not yet been released, so I was blessed to have a gynecologist who heard me say, "I have this odd pain on my left side." Her action started me on the road toward diagnosis and a visit to a gynecologic oncologist. The year I was diagnosed, I was one of roughly 700 women diagnosed with this disease in New Jersey. Not a huge number, but if you include all those people impacted by the disease as well as their family and friends, the number is much larger.

The journey is not an easy one. Hearing that you have ovarian cancer makes you weak in the knees and takes your breath away. You think of the road that lies ahead—chemotherapy, losing your hair, losing the organs that brought (or could bring) your children into the world—and you allow yourself to think the unthinkable: that you might not make it. And you sink a bit further toward the ground.

That is when somehow you find the strength to tackle whatever the disease throws at you and you start standing a bit straighter. Many people have asked me how I was able to deal with cancer. I tell them I would not have been able to do it if not for my family and friends, my faith, good medicine, and wonderful doctors. You find support from loving family and friends who bring you food, join you at treatment sessions, and help you with chores.

Then you look further, and you find others diagnosed with ovarian cancer. They tell you how their toes feel "big"—the same feeling you had when you were young and spent too much time out in the snow (a friend's way of describing neuropathy). Others explain to you why your nose is constantly running (hair loss includes those tiny ones in your nose, too.) When you tell them your scalp hurt as your hair fell out, they tell you they felt the same way. They complain about not being able to find the right words because of "chemo brain" and you cry together because you found someone who understands your frustration. When they tell you how anxious they are waiting to hear scan results, you can relate exactly to how they feel. You hug each other when you lose one of your "Teal Sisters" (teal is the ovarian cancer awareness color). And when you share others' reactions to your diagnosis (which I describe as the "Oh no... not the disease Gilda Radner had" look), they've seen the same reactions too. These women "get it." Not every woman diagnosed with ovarian cancer has the same chemotherapy and surgery side effects, but I hope all the women who read this book will be able to make connections with other survivors for the emotional support that is so important in our lives.

I write this book as a survivor who is NED (No Evidence of Disease). I may still suffer from some of the side effects of all the treatments I have had, and I still get nervous before a scan or blood test, but I am thriving in my "new normal." Part of what helps me stay calm is to be prepared. I think of myself as a research "hound," reading journal articles about clinical trials, new treatments, and precision medicine. In this way, I will have the knowledge to make the best treatment decision for whatever lies ahead in the years to come.

I am so happy to see the increase in awareness of ovarian cancer symptoms over the past 10 years. Strong advocacy for the funding of ovarian cancer research by national organizations such as the Ovarian Cancer National Alliance has seen the approval of many of the treatments Dr. Dizon writes about in this edition. There is more work to do, but there are many researchers and gynecologic oncologists dedicating their lives to finding a cure—and this gives me hope.

I dedicate this book to my husband, Nick, who has been with me on this cancer journey from the start. He has been by my side for two surgeries (four if you count the surgeries to insert and remove my port-a-cath), 15 chemotherapy treatments (nine on initial diagnosis and six on recurrence), 20 CT scans, two PET scans, and countless doctor's appointments and blood draws. Without his support and love, I would have surely stopped at chemo number six.

I also dedicate this book to my children, Theresa and Matthew, who make me laugh, take me on adventures to other states and countries, and urge me try new things as I find my new normal. To their spouses, thank you for your support and love for them and me. And to my grandsons, John and Thomas, thank you for the immeasurable joy you have brought me.

I am forever grateful for the outstanding care provided by my "life-savers," Dr. Darlene Gibbon and Dr. Lorna Rodriguez, gynecologic oncologists at Rutgers Cancer

Institute of New Jersey. Thank you, Dr. Gibbon, for launching my advocacy work by recommending I apply to the LiveSTRONG Survivor's Summit in 2006. I am also thankful for the compassionate care provided by the adult oncology treatment nurses, the advance practice nurses in the gynecologic oncology department, and the social workers at the Rutgers Cancer Institute of New Jersey.

Finally, thank you, Dr. Don Dizon, for providing me the opportunity to share my voice with others.

Dorinda "Dee" Sparacio
February 2015

Preface

It has been nine years since the second edition was published in 2006. In that time, we have seen changes in how we classify and treat this disease, as we work towards a more precise and individualized approach to treatment. The important and still highly relevant contributions of my friend and colleague, Nadeem Abu-Rustum, remain embedded in this edition. After re-reading them in preparation of this edition, I still see their value for my own patients and for their loved ones. It remains my hope that the information contained in this book will aid in alleviating some of the uncertainty and confusion felt by many patients and their families who are overwhelmed with information during their diagnosis and subsequent treatment.

As in 2006, life has changed much since the prior edition. I have moved institutions once more; I said goodbye to Providence and the Program in Women's Oncology at Women & Infants' Hospital of Rhode Island. Now, I am at the Massachusetts General Hospital and Harvard Medical School, proud and honored to have been named a Clinical Co-Director of the multidisciplinary Gynecologic Oncology program. Personally, I welcomed twins into my family, and said goodbye to my father, who passed away of heart disease in 2010. All of these serve as reminders that life constantly evolves, no matter what we are faced with at any one point in time.

As in prior editions, this book is for those with ovarian cancer, and their families, friends, significant others, and loved ones, I hope this book will serve as a resource on practical questions regarding the disease. Those of us who treat ovarian cancer like to think we are doing more than performing surgery or administering chemotherapy or radiation. Every day, women welcome me into their lives and, in the process, I get to know them and their families. It is much more than just treatment; it is a relationship that we all hope will extend through the years. The fact is: We can cure ovarian cancer, but even when we cannot, we can help you live with it, too.

I would like to thank my own family for their constant support, including Henry W. Stoll; our children, Isabelle, Harrison and Sophia; my mother, Millionita Dizon; my mother-in-law, Marilyn Z. Stoll; and my four sisters, Michelle, Maerica, Precy, and Marie. Furthermore, I want to give a word of thanks to the Gynecologic Oncology program at the MGH Cancer Center, and my mentor, Michael J. Birrer. Thank you all for your support and the opportunities. Lastly, continued gratitude to my dad, Modesto M. Dizon. Although you are gone, you will never be forgotten.

Don S. Dizon, MD, FACP
January 2015

PART ONE

The Basics

Where are my ovaries? What do they do?

What does it mean to have cancer?

What is a cyst? Is it related to ovarian cancer?
How do a complex ovarian cyst and
a simple cyst differ?

More. . .

1. Where are my ovaries? What do they do?

An understanding of basic female anatomy and the function of the ovaries is a good starting point for the following discussion of ovarian cancer.

The ovaries, fallopian tubes, and uterus are what make up a woman's internal female reproductive organs (**Figure 1**). These organs lie deep in the pelvis and are connected to one another. The cervix is the external extension of the uterus and, together with the vagina and vulva, forms the female external genital tract.

Each woman is born with two ovaries, located on either side of the pelvis and flanking the uterus. Other organs are located near your ovaries: the small bowel and the **omentum**; the bladder, which sits on top of the uterus; and the rectum, which lies under the uterus.

The ovaries are where eggs are stored. The ovaries start to release eggs when girls reach adolescence, and their bodies prepare themselves for possible pregnancy by the release of hormones called **estrogen** and progesterone. Eggs are released at monthly intervals (called **ovulation**), and their release begins the menstrual cycle.

The ovaries are essential as the home to those eggs until they're released into the fallopian tube and travel to the uterus. If an egg is not fertilized, the uterus sheds its lining. This process is manifest as **menstruation**, or your period. The ovaries not only carry a woman's eggs, but also are responsible for the release of estrogen which causes breast development and other sexual characteristics in women.

Omentum

Fatty apron that drapes from the stomach and colon.

Estrogen

A female hormone produced by the ovaries; it is responsible for female changes during maturity.

Ovulation

Process of egg release from the ovary.

Menstruation

Vaginal bleeding due to endometrial shedding following ovulation when the egg is not fertilized.

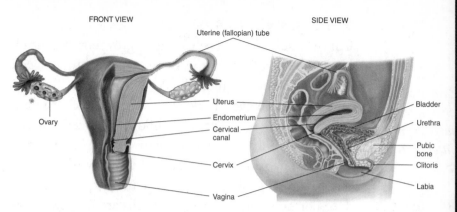

Figure 1 Anatomy of the female reproductive system. Reproduced from Alters S, *Biology: Understanding Life, Third Edition.* © 1999 Jones and Bartlett Publishers, Inc., Sudbury, MA.

As a woman ages, the ovaries slowly stop producing hormones, which results in **menopause**. During menopause, the process of egg release slows down and eventually stops. In addition, estrogen production also slows. The uterus responds to changes in hormone levels and doesn't build up as much tissue as it used to, causing periods to become irregular until they, too, eventually stop. The symptoms of menopause occur owing to the gradual decline in the levels of estrogen produced by the ovaries.

Menopause

Physical changes marking the end of a woman's fertile years, the most notable change being the cessation of menstrual cycles.

2. What does it mean to have cancer?

As they do with other organs, a number of diseases and malfunctions can affect the ovaries. Cancer is just one of these. As we get into the discussion of ovarian cancer, we'll describe some common diseases that can be associated with, or sometimes confused with, ovarian cancer, such as ovarian cysts and borderline **tumors** (see Question 3 on page 6 and Question 4 on page 9). First, however, it is most important that you understand what cancer is—and what it is not.

Tumor

A mass of cells that grow abnormally.

WHAT CANCER IS

Cancer results when a cell starts to grow out of control. Normally, cells follow the same cycle of growth, cell division, and eventual death. When we were still developing, first as babies inside our mothers and continuing on while we were infants and children, our cells rapidly grew and divided. The end result was **differentiation**—it's what enabled a red blood cell to carry oxygen, an intestinal cell to absorb food, and an ovary cell to produce hormones to make eggs. If cells are injured or get too old, they undergo a process called **apoptosis**, or programmed cell death. This is what keeps us healthy and all our organs operating normally.

Some of our organs keep the ability to divide in order to replace dead and dying cells. These include the skin, gastrointestinal tract, hair follicles, and to a large degree, the ovaries, which replace their surface after an egg is released.

If a cell undergoes changes in its building blocks, called DNA, it can escape this tightly regulated life cycle. These DNA changes, also called mutations, can allow cells to keep growing and dividing. They no longer respond to your body's signals to stop dividing, and this process of unchecked cell division results in a mass of such cells, called a tumor. If a tumor cell breaks free from its origin (in this case, the ovarian cell within the ovary) it can travel through the bloodstream and land in another area of one's body far away (in the lung, for example) and start growing there; it is by definition **metastatic**. These two features—unchecked cell growth and the ability to metastasize—define cancer.

Cancer results when a cell starts to grow out of control.

Differentiation

The process of cells maturing so they can perform specific processes in our bodies.

Apoptosis

Programmed cell death.

Metastatic

Adjective used to describe a tumor that has spread.

WHAT CANCER ISN'T

It's important to state at this point that cancer is not something that can be passed from one person to another, like a virus or bacteria; cancer is not an infectious disease. You can't get cancer from another person, nor can you give it to someone else by simply coming into contact with that person, even close contact. A lot of factors contribute to the development of cancer, and having a family history of cancer is one of them. However, even if your mother had ovarian cancer, it doesn't mean that you will certainly also develop cancer—although you might have a higher risk of getting it than someone whose mother did not have it. Most important, cancer is not an automatic death sentence. That's a reaction many people have because, for decades, we lacked effective treatments for most kinds of cancers, and significant fear and stigma were attached to cancer. Thankfully, medicine has come a long way, and although cancer is still a fearsome thing, many people survive it, and some are completely cured. Innovations in treatment and new drugs are developed continually, so that even the most dangerous forms of cancer are becoming increasingly curable as new information about how cancer works is uncovered.

Cancer is not an automatic death sentence.

HOW CANCER SPREADS

Cancer can spread in three ways: by extending into surrounding tissue; by passing through the blood supply, a process called hematogenous dissemination; or by traveling in the **lymphatic system**, the "cleaning system" of the body, in a process termed **lymphatic spread**. Knowing the ways in which cancers spread is important, because such knowledge is often used to decide what type of surgery is necessary and what other types of treatment are necessary (such as the use of chemotherapy and the number of cycles needed).

Lymphatic system

A network of lymphatic channels, lymph nodes, and organs, such as the spleen and the tonsils, that forms the major component of the immune system.

Lymphatic spread

Metastasis of cancer cells through the lymphatic system.

THE BASICS

Peritoneum

The lining of the peritoneal cavity.

Colon

The large intestine, part of your gastrointestinal tract. Its function is to absorb water and food and to excrete stool.

Peritoneal seeding

The process of cancer spreading to involve the peritoneal surface.

Carcinomatosis

Cancer deposits along the abdomen, often along the bowel and involving the omentum.

Computed tomography (CT)

Otherwise known as a CT scan, this is a highly sensitive radiology exam used to help diagnose and follow patients with cancer.

Septations

Thin membranes or walls dividing an area into multiple chambers. Often used to describe complex cysts seen on ultrasound.

Anechoic

Used in ultrasound studies, describes a lack of different ultrasound signals, commonly seen with simple cysts.

In the case of ovarian cancer, cells that line the ovary acquire genetic mutations that enable them to become cancer. Unlike many other cancers that tend to spread throughout the body, ovarian cancer prefers the environment within the abdominal cavity (also termed the **peritoneum**). Although it can spread to the liver and lungs or to other places, ovarian cancer is more commonly found growing within the pelvis or, when more advanced, in the abdomen. There, it can land anywhere around the abdominal cavity, surrounding the small bowel or **colon**, as a process called **peritoneal seeding** or **carcinomatosis**. These features are used in the staging (or classification) system for ovarian cancer (discussed in Question 17 on page 29).

3. What is a cyst? Is it related to ovarian cancer? How does a complex ovarian cyst and a simple cyst differ?

A cyst is defined as a fluid-filled growth. Most cysts are not cancer and will go away if left on their own. Ovarian cysts are very common in women before menopause; however, they can also be seen after menopause. On the basis of how they look under ultrasound, **computed tomography (CT)**, or magnetic resonance imaging (MRI), cysts can be one of two types: simple ovarian cysts or complex ovarian cysts.

Simple ovarian cysts are generally thin-walled and contain fluid. As seen on ultrasound, they have a characteristic appearance: They're bland, with a uniform wall around them; they do not have walls within them (also called **septations**); and they do not have differences in their internal appearance (also called **anechoic**). They're common and occur during egg formation, or ovulation.

When an egg forms, it forms in a follicle. If this follicle becomes big enough, it can be seen by ultrasound as a cyst (**Figure 2**); in this situation, they are often termed functional cysts. Cysts appearing this way are generally not cancerous.

Complex ovarian cysts are defined by the presence of internal walls within the cyst (septations) leading to the appearance of different rooms within the cyst (**multi-compartmental**), different appearances within the cyst (**echogenic**), the appearance of buds in the cyst cavity (**papilla**), or differences in the thickness of the surrounding wall (**Figure 3**). Complex ovarian cyst walls may be thicker; they may show nodularity, a solid component, or debris. Complex cysts are more of a concern. They may be associated with cancer, particularly after menopause. Additionally, with special ultrasound imaging to assess blood flow (called Doppler imaging), these complex cysts may be found to be vascular, which may also raise concerns about the possibility of cancer.

Multi-compartmental

Multiple spaces, used to describe a finding seen in complex cysts on imaging studies, like ultrasounds.

Echogenic

An ultrasound term describing complex patterns seen within a cyst.

Papilla

Budding formations on structures, seen on ultrasound or other imaging.

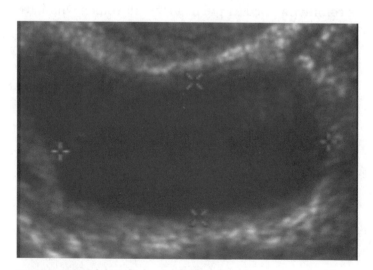

Figure 2 Ultrasound image of a single ovarian cyst.

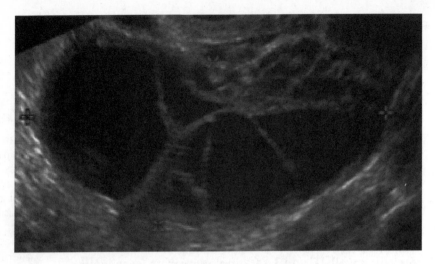

Figure 3 Ultrasound image of a complex ovarian cyst.

The features of the cyst can best be determined by imaging studies, such as a pelvic ultrasound or a pelvic MRI. Depending on the features of the cyst as seen by imaging studies and on other clinical factors, a surgeon will make a decision with a patient as to whether to observe this cyst or to remove it surgically. Observation is commonly used in premenopausal women who have simple cysts or complex cysts that appear to be caused by hemorrhage or bleeding in the ovary, a common occurrence with ovulation.

Surgery is usually considered for large simple cysts that may cause symptoms of pain; for complex cysts with any of the previously discussed findings (papilla, multicompartmental, or thick-walled) at any age; or for complex cysts after menopause. Obtaining a blood tumor marker level, such as that obtained by CA-125 (see Question 15 on page 26) may be helpful, but the test cannot specifically identify ovarian cancer.

4. What is a tumor? How do benign and malignant tumors differ?

A tumor is a mass of abnormal cells. To be specific, the term *tumor* is not synonymous with cancer. You can develop tumors that aren't cancerous, termed benign. The main difference between a **benign** tumor and a malignant tumor is that benign tumors do not spread.

In fact, most epithelial ovarian tumors are benign. Examples of these are **adenomas**. However, if a tumor can spread and invade, it is no longer benign and is considered to be malignant. A malignant tumor is synonymous with cancer. Pathologists refer to malignant tumors as carcinomas. The malignant counterparts to the previously mentioned adenomas are **adenocarcinomas**, which are the most common type of ovarian cancer.

5. What is a borderline tumor? Is it ovarian cancer, or isn't it?

Some women go to their doctor with signs and symptoms of ovarian cancer, undergo surgery to remove the cancer, and then are told, "Don't worry about it; it wasn't cancer after all, it was a **borderline** tumor." This often results in more confusion and questions than even before the surgery.

Borderline tumors of the ovary do not appear normal through the microscope but do not have the appearance of cancer, either. They show evidence of increased growth and changes in their architecture that may not be considered normal to a pathologist. However, they differ from ovarian cancer because they do not show evidence of invasion into the surrounding ovarian tissue.

THE BASICS

Benign
Not cancerous.

Adenomas
Noncancerous tumors arising from epithelial cells.

Adeno-carcinomas
Type of cancer, arising from the cells of epithelial origin.

You can develop tumors that aren't cancerous, termed benign.

Borderline
A term used to describe a tumor that does not appear normal but does not meet a pathologist's criteria for cancer; otherwise described as low malignant potential.

Therefore, they're placed in an intermediate-risk group of tumors, which is why they're called borderline or are said to have low malignant potential. They are not, strictly speaking, ovarian cancer, but they're nevertheless an abnormality in the ovaries that can be harmful and must be treated.

Borderline tumors account for approximately 15% of all ovarian tumors. They require surgical staging just as ovarian cancers do. Although, by their very definition, they are not invasive, they do have the potential to deposit throughout the abdominal cavity, which is why they require **surgical staging**. In fact, their stage (see Question 18 on page 30 and Table 4 on page 31) appears to be an important predictor of survival and recurrence.

Surgical staging

Procedure of determining the extent of cancer present.

Stage I patients are likely to be cured at surgery, whereas those with more advanced disease are at greater risk of recurrence. Still, the prognosis of women with borderline tumors is quite good, with more than 85% of patients alive 5 years after diagnosis.

6. What is a dermoid cyst?

A dermoid cyst is the more common name of a mature teratoma, which is a specific type of germ-cell tumor (discussed in Question 8 on page 14). Dermoid cysts are the most common type of tumor in young women and commonly present as an ovarian mass. They arise when a cell destined to become an egg starts to divide within your ovary, rather than dividing and growing in your uterus after it's fertilized. In the process of developing, such cells may also grow into different tissue types, such as teeth, hair, and even lung tissue. Cancer arising from a dermoid cyst is very rare, especially if it occurs in women below the age of 40, and surgery to remove the mass is all that's usually needed. Most women can expect to be cured after surgical removal of this tumor.

7. What is a Krukenberg tumor?

It might be confusing to be told that you have a cancerous growth in your ovaries, but you don't have ovarian cancer. The reason for this strange fact is that a type of cancer is always defined by where it started, not where it's found, which means that lung cancer found in the bones is still lung cancer, and breast cancer found in the liver is still breast cancer. This is important because different forms of cancer are treated with different methods: Chemotherapy drugs that work against lung cancer, for instance, may not work as well against breast cancer or ovarian cancer, and vice versa. A **Krukenberg tumor** is cancer that's found in the ovary but started in the gastrointestinal tract, typically in the stomach. Because these tumors arise from somewhere other than the ovary, Krukenberg tumors technically are not ovarian cancer; this term is reserved for cancer that begins in the ovary. Treatment of a Krukenberg tumor is dictated by where it came from originally, so the treatments described in this book probably do not apply to patients with Krukenberg tumors.

Because these tumors arise from somewhere other than the ovary, Krukenberg tumors technically are not ovarian cancer.

THE BASICS

Krukenberg tumor

A cancer that has gone into the ovary from another place, usually starting in the stomach.

PART TWO

Risk Factors, Diagnosis, and Staging of Ovarian Cancer

What does it mean to have ovarian cancer?

Are there risk factors for ovarian cancer?

Is hormone replacement therapy associated with ovarian cancer?

More...

8. What does it mean to have ovarian cancer?

Along with the uterus and fallopian tubes, the ovaries comprise the internal female gynecological tract. As discussed in Question 1 on page 2, the ovaries have two main functions: (1) the release of hormones that regulate menstruation and pregnancy and (2) the storage of eggs. Every time an egg is released, the ovary must repair itself and undergoes a process called **regeneration**, in which the surface is rebuilt.

Regeneration
To grow back.

The ovary is composed of three different cell types, or histology: surface or epithelial tissue; germ cells, which produce eggs; and stromal tissue, the mesh that supports the ovary. All three tissue types can give rise to ovarian cancer, but not all such cancers are treated the same way. This book focuses primarily on the treatment of the epithelial ovarian cancers, unless otherwise stated. **Table 1** lists the types of nonepithelial ovarian cancer.

Mixed mesodermal tumors
Tumors of dual origin with one part consisting of carcinomas and the other part consisting of sarcoma, hence their other designation as a carcinosarcoma.

Other types of ovarian cancer can occur beyond these, but they're much rarer. These types include **mixed mesodermal tumors** (or carcinosarcomas) and small-cell cancers. The different types of cancer underscore the importance of tissue analysis by a pathologist.

Table 1 Nonepithelial Ovarian Cancer

Histology	Percentage of All Ovarian Tumors
Metastatic	5–6%
Sex cord/stromal	5–8%
Germ-cell tumors	3%
Mixed mesodermal tumors	< 1%
Lymphoma	< 1%

Epithelial ovarian cancer is the most common type of ovarian cancer. It is a cancer that occurs in the surface (epithelium) of the ovaries and, as discussed in Question 9 on page 18, is related to the frequency of ovulation. Recent developments into the origin of ovarian cancer suggest that the fallopian tube may be where most ovarian cancers arise from. While there is no practical implications of this as far as the treatment of ovarian cancer is concerned today, it may have implications on how we can help prevent ovarian cancer without having to remove the ovaries. This topic is further discussed in Question 90 on page 132.

Although women of any age can develop ovarian cancer, most commonly it's diagnosed in women older than 60. Estimates claim that more than 25,000 women each year will be diagnosed with this cancer. Epithelial ovarian cancers can be classified further on the basis of the type of cells seen through a microscope. The classifications are serous (most common), mucinous, endometrioid, transitional-cell, and clear-cell types of epithelial ovarian cancers. If a cancer bears no resemblance to any of these types of cancers, is it termed **undifferentiated**. The type of epithelial cancer generally does not alter the treatment plan, although clear-cell cancer may not respond as well as the others to chemotherapy.

Germ-cell tumors arise from the cells that produce eggs. Most germ-cell tumors are diagnosed in young women and make up 20% of all ovarian tumors, of which 3% are malignant. In 90% of cases, they involve only one ovary. Given that these tumors tend to appear in young women who may want to have children at some time, sparing the unaffected ovary is a high-priority.

Undifferentiated

A pathologist's term to describe cellular changes of a cancer cell; this describes cells that bear no resemblance at all to normal cells.

Table 2 lists the different types of germ-cell tumors. The most common type of germ-cell tumor is the dysgerminoma, which represents 50% of all germ-cell tumors. The second most common is the **endodermal sinus**, or yolk-sac tumor. The immature teratoma is the third most common, and **prognosis** with these is highly dependent on what they look like under the microscope; they are graded as low or high grade by a pathologist, based on the amount of early nerve tissue seen in the tumor itself. Approximately 10% of germ-cell tumors will be made up of various types of tissue and are called mixed germ-cell tumors.

The type of germ-cell tumor that the pathologist finds under the microscope is a crucial factor in determining whether chemotherapy is used after surgery. Women who have had a thorough surgical evaluation and are found to have stage I dysgerminoma or a low-grade immature teratoma do not require chemotherapy and have an excellent prognosis.

Endodermal sinus tumor

A type of germ-cell tumor, derived from early cells destined to become eggs. Otherwise, they are referred to as yolk-sac tumors.

Prognosis

An estimate of the outlook following the diagnosis of a disease such as cancer.

Table 2 Germ-Cell Tumors

Dysgerminoma
Endodermal sinus tumor (or yolk-sac tumor)
Embryonal carcinoma
Polyembryoma
Choriocarcinoma

Teratoma
    mature
    immature

Mixed germ-cell tumor

A lot of work has been done to identify what factors influence prognosis (prospect for recovery) in women with germ-cell tumors. A poor prognosis is associated with mixed-cell-type tumors, with large tumors (greater than 10 centimeters) that are made up of endodermal sinus tumor, with choriocarcinoma, or with immature teratoma. Tumors measuring less than 10 centimeters were found to offer a good prognosis, regardless of cell type.

Ovarian cancers that arise from the surrounding connective tissue of the ovary are called sex cord–stromal tumors. The cells that give rise to these tumors are responsible for the release of female hormones: estrogen (in the case of Sertoli cell, granulosa cell, and theca cell tumors) and progesterone (in the case of Sertoli-Leydig and steroid cell tumors). Sex cord–stromal tumors account for 5% of all ovarian tumors. The most common type is the granulosa-cell tumor. Because this type of tumor produces hormones, women tend to become symptomatic when the disease is present at an early stage. These tumors can affect both ovaries in 4–26% of cases, which makes a complete surgical evaluation very important.

The overall prognosis for women with sex cord–stromal tumors is very good, particularly because women tend to report to doctors early with these tumors. However, even in cases of early disease, the tumor can come back. It's not uncommon for women to have their cancer return 5 to 20 years after their initial diagnosis, which is why close monitoring of women with such tumors is very important. These tumor cell types are included in **Table 3**.

9. Are there risk factors for ovarian cancer?

Ovarian cancer likely arises from many factors and most likely is due to genetic damage that builds up over time.

As with most other cancers, ovarian cancer likely arises from many factors and most likely is due to genetic damage that builds up over time. It is important to distinguish the difference between "genetic damage" and "hereditary damage" in this context. Changes to one's genes, called mutations, occur spontaneously as a simple, random mistake in cell growth, sometimes related to an environmental factor. Most mutations are harmless; many that are harmful nevertheless do no damage because they are eliminated by the body's immune system, but some are able to escape the immune system, replicate themselves, and form cancers. A small number of these cancer-causing **mutations** can be passed from parent to child. However, most ovarian cancers are not familial or hereditary. Instead, they happen to patients randomly, or as **sporadic** cancers. Hereditary ovarian cancer is discussed more in Question 10, starting on the next page.

Mutations

Genetic changes in DNA; mutations are not always harmful but sometimes can be associated with cancer development.

Sporadic

Isolated; to occur without a pattern.

Several factors are associated with an increased risk for ovarian cancer. The most common type of ovarian

Table 3 Sex Cord–Stromal Tumors

Granulosa-cell tumor
Thecoma-fibroma
Fibroma
Sertoli-Leydig cell
Leydig cell
Sarcomatoid (undifferentiated)
Gynandroblastoma
Unclassified

cancer—epithelial ovarian cancer—appears to be related to how many times a woman ovulates. Every time an egg is released, the ovarian surface has to be repaired; each time this happens, it creates a risk that genetic mutations will accumulate. This condition may lead to epithelial ovarian cancer. This hypothesis is supported by the fact that decreasing ovulation with the use of oral contraceptives is associated with a decreased risk of getting ovarian cancer in the future.

Other risk factors for ovarian cancer include older age and a family history of breast and ovarian cancer. The use of hormone replacement therapy (HRT) is not considered a risk factor (see Question 11 on page 20). The use of fertility drugs for women having trouble becoming pregnant has been debated as a possible risk for increased ovarian cancer, but there is no conclusive evidence that these medications cause ovarian cancer.

10. How does ovarian cancer run in families? What is a BRCA mutation?

Although the majority of ovarian cancer does not run in families (or *sporadic* ovarian cancer), about 15 to 20% of ovarian cancers run in families. This happens because of a genetic mutation that makes women in these families have a higher risk of ovarian cancer than in the general population. This topic is also discussed in Question 93 on page 133.

Among the best characterized are mutations in the breast cancer susceptibility (BRCA) genes. There are two well-characterized BRCA mutations that increase the risk of ovarian cancer (and breast cancer) in women: *BRCA1* and *BRCA2*, and of these, mutations in *BRCA1* carries a greater risk of ovarian cancer than those involving *BRCA2*. By age 70, the estimated risk approaches 40–60% and 15–20%, respectively. How common these mutations are seems to depend on one's ethnicity as well, with higher rates in populations founded by a small ancestral group, once felt to be isolated, either by geography or by culture, known as the **Founder Effect**. Populations with this founder effect (and hence, a high rate of BRCA mutations) include Ashkenazi Jews, French Canadians, Icelanders, and U.S. Hispanics. The specific mutations considered Founder Mutations include the 185delAG and 5382insC mutations of *BRCA1* and the 6174delIT mutation of *BRCA2*.

Founder Effect

Greater inheritance of a genetic mutation in a well-defined population that can theoretically be traced back to a common ancestor.

11. Is hormone replacement therapy associated with ovarian cancer?

Hormone replacement therapy (HRT) has been used in women for several decades as a way to control the symptoms of menopause. The main reason for using HRT is to help women deal with hot flashes and night sweats associated with menopause. Although long-term use of estrogen plus progesterone HRT has been associated with a slightly increased risk of breast cancer, HRT's association with ovarian cancer is less clear.

12. What are the symptoms of ovarian cancer?

The main symptoms of ovarian cancer are bloating, abdominal pain, and distension.

The main symptoms of ovarian cancer are bloating, abdominal pain, and distension. A recent study from the University of California at Irvine compared the prior symptoms and testing of women who were eventually diagnosed with ovarian cancer with those of women who did not have a cancer diagnosis and to a third group of women diagnosed with breast cancer. These researchers showed that the specific symptoms of bloating and abdominal pain were more likely in women diagnosed with ovarian cancer and represented "target symptoms." More importantly, they showed that these symptoms were present as long as 6 months prior to the diagnosis of ovarian cancer. On the basis of this work and prior research like it, we feel a woman should be cautioned that if she develops bloating, an increase in her waistline not due to a change in eating habits, lower abdominal discomfort, or pelvic pain, she should seek consultation with a physician. A work-up should include pelvic imaging and a CA-125, especially if the symptoms are unexplained.

Occasionally, women have shortness of breath that can be misinterpreted as a heart or lung problem; actually, it may be due to a buildup of fluid in the lung (a **pleural effusion**). Acid reflux, constipation, nausea, or vomiting may also be obvious, particularly when associated with early sensations of fullness at meals or a generally decreased appetite.

Pleural effusion

Fluid build-up around the lungs.

Women with germ-cell tumors often go to their doctor with abdominal pain that persists over several days or weeks and are also found to have a palpable (touchable) pelvic mass when examined. If the mass twists on itself or undergoes **torsion**, it can cause immediate and often unbearable pain. Such a mass can also cause pain due to bleeding or if it ruptures. These cancers typically grow very rapidly and at surgery can be as large as 40 centimeters. Fortunately, 70% of women with germ-cell tumors will be diagnosed with early-stage disease.

Torsion

Act of twisting or turning in on itself (ovarian torsion, for example).

Sex cord–stromal tumors appear early owing to their production of hormones, and their appearance can range from early puberty in young girls to postmenopausal bleeding in mature women. Abnormal vaginal bleeding is a common reason for women with granulosa-cell tumors to see their doctor. Other ways the disease can show up is by a mass felt on physical examination, ovarian torsion, rupture, or hemorrhage. Thecomas (tumors of theca cells) actively secrete hormones, and women seek a doctor owing to the effects of too much estrogen. Women with Sertoli-cell tumors also go to their doctor for the same reason, although they may have high blood pressure from excess production of a kidney hormone—called **renin**—necessary for blood pressure regulation. Fifty percent of women with Sertoli-Leydig-cell tumors notice symptoms related to too many androgens, or male hormones, which can cause a decrease in breast tissue or male-pattern baldness.

Renin

A hormone released by the kidney normally that is important in maintaining hydration.

Dee's comment:

During my annual visit with my gynecologist in 2005, I mentioned to her an odd pain I was having on the left side of my abdomen. I thought it was just a pulled muscle. I had also put on some weight but I assumed that the weight gain had to do with my metabolism slowing down as I aged.

After explaining how I felt to my gynecologist, she thought it best to send me for a transvaginal ultrasound. The day after the ultrasound I was in the emergency room in severe pain. That visit led to an MRI that showed my ovaries had doubled in size. I was then referred to Dr. Lorna Rodriguez, a gynecologic oncologist at Rutgers Cancer Institute of New Jersey, a NCI Comprehensive Cancer Center. She and Dr. Darlene Gibbon, also a gynecologic oncologist, performed surgery and administered chemotherapy.

Over the past 10 years many national and local ovarian cancer organizations have helped to raise awareness of the symptoms of the disease—bloating, pain, frequent urination, feeling full quickly, and pelvic or abdominal pain. Until a screening test for ovarian cancer is developed, knowledge of the symptoms is so very important for all women.

13. What is ascites? What causes it? How do you treat it?

Ascites is the build-up of fluid in the **peritoneal cavity**. The peritoneum is a sac made of a thin layer of tissue that lines the abdominal cavity and covers most of our internal abdominal and pelvic organs and the intestines. Ascites is a hallmark of advanced ovarian carcinoma, and it is very commonly seen in patients with disease that has spread outside of the ovary to involve the peritoneum or other organs in the abdomen. Ascites can develop for numerous reasons; however, in the setting of ovarian cancer, the most likely explanation is the spread of disease to organs inside the abdomen, the omentum, and the diaphragm. Ascites may be formed due to non-cancerous conditions such as liver disease or heart failure, but in the setting of ovarian cancer, ascites is most commonly considered "malignant ascites." Ascites may accumulate to a large volume; some patients may have several liters of this usually amber-colored fluid inside the abdomen, which causes distention and may be the presenting symptom of ovarian carcinoma. Women with ascites may complain of discomfort, indigestion, and sometimes difficulty breathing due to pressure on the diaphragm.

Treatment of ascites usually consists of a combination of a drainage procedure followed by chemotherapy. A drainage of the ascites can be performed by **paracentesis**, a bedside procedure done under a local anesthetic to the abdominal wall. A small needle is introduced through the

Ascites
Fluid build-up within the abdomen.

Peritoneal cavity
The abdominal space.

Paracentesis
The process of removing ascites.

skin into the peritoneal cavity and connected to a vacuum bottle, where the fluid is drained from the abdomen.

Several liters of fluid can be removed this way with almost immediate symptom relief. Ascites also can be drained at the time of a surgical procedure for the cancer. However, if the patient does not receive chemotherapy promptly, ascites is very likely to reaccumulate within several days. The majority of patients with new ovarian cancer (70–80%) will respond to chemotherapy, and chemotherapy will usually prevent reaccumulation of ascites. Chemotherapy can be given either intravenously or sometimes through a semi-permanent catheter, called an **intraperitoneal port**, that is placed into the peritoneal cavity where chemotherapy washes are given directly into the peritoneum.

Intraperitoneal port

A device surgically placed under the skin and into the abdomen that allows directed treatment into the abdomen.

If the cancer does not respond to initial chemotherapy or returns after some time and starts to grow once more, your belly may fill up with ascites again. In that event, doctors use other types of chemotherapy to get control of your cancer, which is the primary way to control the ascites. If the swelling continues to recur, your physician may repeat the paracentesis multiple times.

14. What about pleural effusions? How do you treat them?

A pleural effusion is the build-up of fluid within the lung cavity, which is lined by a thin membrane of tissue called the pleura that envelops the lungs and the inner lining of the chest wall. Pleural effusions are occasionally seen with cases of advanced ovarian carcinoma. Like ascites, pleural effusions may be related to other medical conditions such as inflammation, infection, or heart disease. In the setting of advanced ovarian cancer, it may be an extension of advanced ascites related to advanced stage cancer. A large pleural effusion may cause shortness of breath and sometimes causes difficulty breathing (**dyspnea**).

The treatment of a pleural effusion will depend on the size of the effusion and the patient's symptoms. A moderate or large symptomatic pleural effusion that is causing symptoms of shortness of breath will usually require drainage. This procedure, called a **thoracentesis**, can be performed as a bedside procedure. A needle is introduced under local anesthesia between the ribs to aspirate the fluid from the chest and allow the lung tissue to expand and provide more room for breathing. This will usually result in immediate and significant improvement in breathing and less discomfort to the patient.

Alternatively, a pleural effusion can also be treated by placement of a chest tube by an **interventional radiologist** or a thoracic surgeon. A small incision is made between the ribs and a small tube is introduced into the chest cavity and connected to a special suction device; this drains the fluid from the pleural cavity continuously and allows re-expansion of the lung over several days. The advantage of chest tube placement is that it allows the drainage of a large amount of effusion over several days. It also allows the clinician who performed the procedure the chance to introduce a chemical substance into the lung for a procedure called **pleurodesis**, where a chemical substance such as talc is used to seal the pleura and hopefully prevent reaccumulation of malignant pleural effusion in the future.

Similar to malignant ascites in the peritoneal cavity, the ultimate treatment for a malignant pleural effusion will be effective systemic chemotherapy that will reduce the

Dyspnea
Shortness of breath.

Thoracentesis
Procedure of draining a pleural effusion.

interventional radiologist
A radiologist skilled in performing procedures guided by imaging.

Pleurodesis
Process performed to prevent further build-up of fluid around the lung.

bulk of the tumor or completely eliminate the tumor. This will provide the patient with the best likelihood of the fluid not reaccumulating in the future.

15. What tests are used to diagnose ovarian cancer? How is a cancer diagnosis determined from these tests?

Ovarian cancer is diagnosed at surgery. Prior to surgery, tests that may help to make the diagnosis include a pelvic ultrasound (to check the size and nature of the ovaries) and a CT scan of the abdomen and pelvis. Such a scan can show a pelvic mass and also describe the presence of ascites (fluid buildup) and the possibility of **peritoneal carcinomatosis** or liver involvement. An MRI (magnetic resonance imaging) of the pelvis is also helpful to describe the nature of any pelvic abnormality, especially how deeply involved a tumor is with its surroundings.

The main diagnostic tool for ovarian cancer, however, remains surgery. All the imaging tests described previously can suggest ovarian cancer. However, the tumor has to be removed, seen under a microscope, and examined by a pathologist to confirm the diagnosis.

To make a diagnosis of cancer, a pathologist looks for specific features in a cell. Some of the criteria that influence a decision are (1) changes in the cell that make it appear different from a normal appearance, otherwise known as **atypia**; (2) intact or distorted architecture of the cell; and (3) evidence that the cell is dividing actively, also known as **mitosis**. A pathologist can also look for evidence of spread, or **metastases**, through the microscope by examining other tissue, such as the lymph nodes.

Peritoneal carcinomatosis

Involvement of the omentum or bowels with cancer, usually the size of "rice granules" or tumor nodules.

Atypia

Used by pathologists, it describes abnormal cellular changes seen under the microscope.

Mitosis

Process of cells dividing.

Metastases

Tumor that has spread to distant places in the body.

A pathologist looking at an ovarian tumor may see the cancer cells starting to pass through blood channels (**capillaries**) or lymph channels within the tissue; that may signal an increased risk for metastasis. In some instances, the pathologist can make a diagnosis of cancer without needing to look at the tumor. If fluid was surrounding the lung (pleural effusion) or was present within the abdomen (ascites), analyzing the fluid for cancer cells (known as **cytology**) could be sufficient to make a diagnosis of cancer.

Capillaries

The smallest blood vessels within your body.

Cytology

The process of examining cells under the microscope; the sample is usually obtained from floating cells in the fluid of the abdomen (ascites) or chest (pleural effusions).

16. What is the CA-125 test, and what is its purpose?

The CA-125 is a blood test that can be used in the management of ovarian cancer. However, it cannot be used to make a diagnosis of ovarian cancer. The CA-125 is a glycoprotein, meaning a protein with a carbohydrate molecule attached to it (hence the CA, which stands for carbohydrate **antigen**).

Antigen

A protein that sits on or is released from cells that can be targeted with an antibody or a vaccine.

"Normal" CA-125 varies from woman to woman, so the measurement isn't an absolute, and fluctuations in the CA-125 level are common: It might be elevated during one doctor's visit but be below normal 4 weeks later. Such changes in the CA-125 suggest that other factors not related to ovarian cancer—such as endometriosis, pelvic inflammatory disease, and uterine fibroids, to name a few—can influence the CA-125 level. The CA-125 level is useful to help follow women who are being treated or have been treated for ovarian cancer and whose CA-125 was high at the time of diagnosis. That is, the levels of this antigen compared to previous measurements can be used as an indicator of what might be happening with the patient's ovarian cancer. If the

CA-125 results remain low and within normal limits, it's usually a good sign that the disease is not back or growing. However, if the CA-125 value starts to rise beyond what the laboratory considers a normal value (in most labs, < 35 mg/dL), a recurrence must be ruled out. Nevertheless, the CA-125 is not, and should not be, the only measurement for such tracking (or follow-up) in ovarian cancer.

The CA-125 may also be used in the initial evaluation of an ovarian cyst. A normal CA-125 result is often reassuring and may help your doctor decide to observe—as opposed to operate on—an ovarian cyst. However, if the CA-125 result is elevated, it may be evidence that your doctor uses to recommend that an ovarian cyst be surgically evaluated.

Remember that the CA-125 (as mentioned) is not a test specific only to ovarian cancer, and its results can be elevated in a variety of noncancerous conditions, such as endometriosis, uterine fibroids, inflammatory diseases, other cancers such as breast or lung cancer, and even menstruation. This limits the use of CA-125 in ovarian cancer screening.

Dee's comment:

If you are recently diagnosed or in treatment and reading this book, I want to warn you that you may find yourself stressing about your CA-125 results. When I was in treatment after diagnosis I could never receive my results fast enough, and I would worry a few days before the test and while I wait for the results. Over time, though, that anxiety is less and less.

When I recurred in 2008, my CA-125 result was 17, within the normal range of the test. For a year prior, my CA-125 results had been stable at 13. Even though my CA-125 was normal, a CT scan showed disease on my liver and spleen. Since that time, my gynecologic oncologist and I follow the CA-125 trend, not the absolute value of the result.

As long as I feel good and am not experiencing any other symptoms (the same symptoms you have for an initial diagnosis), I don't really worry what my actual CA-125 number is. If it does go up a bit, I am comfortable waiting a month and having the test redone before conducting other tests.

In other cases, oncologists may choose to begin treating a patient's rising CA-125, but my doctor and I have agreed to wait until there is evidence on a scan or if I develop symptoms before beginning treatment.

17. Should I have a PET scan?

A PET (positron emission tomography) scan is a test that allows doctors to evaluate metabolic processes, and most commonly tracks glucose (sugar) metabolism. When cells become cancerous, there can be a detectable increase in their use of glucose, making PET a potentially valuable tool in the evaluation, staging, and tracking of cancer. It is used in the management of multiple tumors including breast, lung, and colorectal cancers. Its role in ovarian cancer continues to be explored and we do not routinely use it in women with ovarian cancer.

Small studies suggest that PET scans can predict response as early as 2 weeks into treatment with chemotherapy, but these results have yet to be tested in larger groups of women.

Whether or not a PET scan is used depends very much on the situation. While not widely used, some clinicians rely on the PET scan to help inform your treatments, while others have not yet adopted it as part of their routine practice. We need better data to help clarify what (if any) role the PET scan has before it should be a part of the routine work-up of women with (or being evaluated for) ovarian cancer.

Dee's comment:

Most of the scans I have had during treatment and follow-up care have been CT (computed tomography) scans. I have had a positron emission tomography (PET) scan during initial treatment. Following nine cycles of chemotherapy, there was one spot on my liver that remained on the CT scan. At that time, my gynecologic oncologist decided that a PET scan would provide information on whether I should continue treatment or stop. By having the PET scan my doctor was able to determine that it was not cancer and that I did not require any more chemotherapy.

18. What is staging? How is ovarian cancer staged?

When you have surgery to remove an ovarian tumor, the surgeon will also check to see whether the cancer has spread throughout the abdomen and pelvis. This process is known as surgical staging (see **Table 4**).

Laparotomy

Surgery through a large incision in the abdomen.

Surgery for ovarian cancer requires a **laparotomy**, a vertical incision in the abdomen starting from the pubic area and extending to the belly button. The surgery requires removal of the omentum, the fatty tissue that drapes between the stomach and colon; removal of lymph nodes from the pelvis and around the largest

Table 4 The 2014 FIGO Staging System of Ovarian Cancer

Stage	Definition
I	Cancer is limited to one or both ovaries.
IA	Cancer is limited to one ovary, and the tumor is confined to the inside of the ovary, without evidence of cancer on the outer surface. No cancerous cells in ascites or pelvic washings.
IB	Cancer is limited to both ovaries without any tumor on their outer surfaces. No cancerous cells in ascites or pelvic washings.
IC	Tumor meets the criteria for either stage IA or stage IB, but one or more of the following are present: spill of fluid at the time of surgery, rupture of the ovarian capsule, tumor involving the surface of the ovary or fallopian tube, or cancerous cells in ascites or pelvic washings.
II	The tumor involves one or both ovaries with extension to other pelvic structures.
IIA	The cancer has extended to and/or involves the uterus and/or the fallopian tubes and/or the ovaries.
IIB	The cancer has extended to other pelvic structures (such as the bladder or rectum).
III	The tumor involves one or both ovaries, and one or both of the following are present: (1) The cancer has spread beyond the pelvis to the lining of the abdomen, or (2) the cancer has spread to the lymph nodes.
IIIA	Cancer has spread to the retroperitoneal nodes and/or metastatic disease involves the abdomen, though only identified under the microscope.
IIIB	Deposits of cancer large enough for the surgeon to see but not exceeding 2 cm in diameter are present in the abdomen (with or without retroperitoneal node involvement).
IIIC	Deposits of cancer exceed 2 cm in diameter and are found in the abdomen (including on the liver or spleen surface, but without extending into the organ itself), with or without retroperitoneal node involvement.
IV	Evidence of distant cancer spread, beyond the abdomen and pelvis.
IVA	Pleural effusion with evidence of cancer cells in the fluid
IVB	Cancer spread to other organs (including the lymph nodes outside the abdominal cavity)

FIGO = Federation International de Gynecologie et d'Obstetrique (International Federation of Gynecologic Oncologists).

Biopsy

Removal of a small amount of tissue for analysis by a pathologist. It can be done during surgery or before surgery using other less invasive procedures.

Bilateral salpingo-oophorectomy

The surgical term for removal of both the right and left fallopian tubes and ovaries.

Total hysterectomy

Surgical excision of the uterus and cervix.

artery in the body, known as the aorta; and obtaining multiple tissue specimens (**biopsies**) from the right and left sides of the pelvis, from the right and left sides of the abdomen, and from both diaphragms. In addition, surgeons would obtain washings from the abdomen to assess for floating cancer cells. The appendix might also be removed. The pelvic part of the procedure requires removal of both tubes and ovaries and the uterus (**bilateral salpingo-oophorectomy** and **total hysterectomy**).

Very few women get ovarian cancer before menopause, so retaining fertility is not a concern for nearly 90% of ovarian cancer patients—but there are occasionally younger women who are diagnosed with cancer before menopause. In selected patients who strongly want to have children some day and in whom no visible disease is seen outside the ovaries at the time of surgery, a fertility-sparing operation could be performed (see Question 27 on page 47).

The staging system is based on the findings at the time of surgery. Table 4 gives the staging system created by the International Federation of Gynecologic Oncologists (FIGO).

19. What is the "grade" of a cancer? Is it the same thing as the "stage"?

Grade

A pathologist term that defines how abnormal a cell is under the microscope.

The **grade** is not the same thing as the stage of a cancer. Staging is a way of describing the location and spread of cancer. The staging system for ovarian cancer requires surgery to determine the extent of disease. The grade of cancer, on the other hand, is a way of describing the cells themselves in comparison to normal cells—a means of saying just how abnormal an abnormal cell appears.

Table 4 describes the staging system in detail. In general, stage I disease is limited to the ovary; stage II cancer will have spread from the ovary to other pelvic organs; stage III cancer has spread to abdominal surfaces, lymph nodes, and intestinal surfaces; and stage IV cancer will have spread to the liver, the lungs, or other distant places. The staging system serves several purposes. First, it provides a standard language so that all of the people involved in treatment of ovarian cancer, from the surgeon to the medical oncologist to the nurses, can understand the extent of disease when a woman presents with ovarian cancer. Second, it is used to decide what kind of treatment is used. Finally, it's used when we try to determine the chances that you may have in beating the cancer (your prognosis).

The grade of a cancer, on the other hand, tells us something quite different. As mentioned in Question 14, the degree of cellular change, or atypia, is an important factor in determining normal from abnormal cells. Pathologists use a scoring system to determine how greatly these cells differ from their normal counterparts; that's termed the grade. In this system, grade I cancers are very similar to normal tissue and are called **well-differentiated**. As cancers look increasingly abnormal, their grade gets higher. Thus, grade II cancers are **moderately differentiated**; grade III cancers are **poorly differentiated**; and grade IV cancers, which bear no resemblance to normal tissue, are **undifferentiated**.

In some cancers, including ovarian cancer, the grade can be used to predict how well your cancer will respond to chemotherapy. Grade I tumors are slow-growing and are not as responsive to chemotherapy, but grade III tumors usually respond well because they are much more active and dividing.

RISK FACTORS, DIAGNOSIS, AND STAGING OF OVARIAN CANCER

Well-differentiated

A pathologist's term to describe cellular changes of a cancer cell; this describes cells that meet the criteria for cancer but still maintain a resemblance to normal cells.

Moderately differentiated

A pathologist's term to describe cellular changes of a cancer cell; cells that do not resemble their normal appearance but are still recognizable as related to their normal counterparts.

Poorly differentiated

A pathologist's term to describe cellular changes of a cancer cell; this describes cells that bear little resemblance to their normal counterparts.

Undifferentiated

A pathologist's term to describe cellular changes of a cancer cell; this describes cells that bear no resemblance at all to normal cells.

20. What is my prognosis, and how is it determined?

A prognosis is an assessment of how a person diagnosed with a specific disease is likely to do and gives an estimate of the likelihood of cure or long-term survival. It is based on the information we have learned over the years about how women with the various stages and grades of ovarian cancer do over time. It is not something that is carved in stone; cancer patients with poor prognoses (i.e., the dreaded statement, "You have six months to live") have been known to do far better than predicted, with some surviving years, even decades, longer than forecast by their prognoses. Every patient is different, and your response to a particular form of treatment may be better or worse than average, so take the prognosis with a grain of salt.

The prognosis of patients with ovarian cancer depends on a variety of factors. Some important factors that have an impact on prognosis are (1) the type of cancer as determined through the microscope, (2) the stage of ovarian cancer, (3) whether all visible cancer was removed at surgery, (4) the size of any disease left after the initial surgery, and (5) your overall medical condition and age.

The prognosis is generally good for stage I ovarian cancer. One recent study indicated that women with stage I ovarian cancer who had a preoperative CA-125 below 30 U/mL and underwent complete surgical evaluation for their disease had a very good prognosis, and may not need further treatment beyond surgery. However, it is still not clear which individual or group of patients can be spared chemotherapy, and a fraction of patients will still require additional treatment in the form of chemotherapy after surgery.

For more advanced stages, the prognosis will depend on the results of the initial surgery. The best surgical result is to leave no visible disease at the end (otherwise known as a **complete resection**). Patients with no visible remaining (residual) disease tend to have a prognosis and overall survival rate better than those of patients whose disease cannot be completely removed. If visible residual disease cannot be completely removed, it is best to leave behind the smallest amount of disease. Patients who have disease less than 1 centimeter in diameter at the end of surgery (otherwise known as **optimal debulking**) do better than those who have disease greater than 1 centimeter (also called a **suboptimal debulking**).

Sometimes in advanced ovarian cancer, a tumor larger than 1 centimeter may be located in close proximity to vital structures, such that attempts to completely remove it would cause significant injury and/or lead to permanent disfigurement or disability. In such cases, surgeons would still require chemotherapy to fight the disease left behind.

Complete resection

Removal of all the tumor in your abdomen and pelvis.

Optimal debulking

Surgical result if residual tumor is less than 1 cm in diameter at the end of surgery.

Suboptimal debulking

Residual disease greater than 1 cm in diameter upon completion of surgery.

21. How does ovarian cancer spread? Does it usually spread to particular locations?

The most dangerous type of ovarian cancer—or any cancer—is cancer that has metastasized, or spread to another part of the body. The danger lies in the fact that once cancer metastasizes, it can go just about anywhere and start growing new tumors. Like other cancers, ovarian cancer that metastasizes can show up in the lungs, liver, or even the brain. However, for reasons not fully understood, this cancer seems to "prefer"

Like other cancers, ovarian cancer that metastasizes can show up in the lungs, liver, or even the brain.

the environment of the abdomen and pelvis and will most often grow and spread in these areas, even when it recurs.

Ovarian cancer can spread (metastasize) in one of three ways. In local extension, the cancer can spread locally, either by growing directly on the surface of adjacent tissue (**direct extension**) or by growing through the surface of the peritoneum, the inner lining of your abdomen. When it spreads by such direct extension, the cancer attaches and then spreads to the fallopian tube, uterus, bladder, peritoneum, or rectal surface. This is a common way for locally advanced disease to spread. The other way is by spreading along the peritoneum. Ovarian cancer can shed from its original site in the ovary and land anywhere on the lining of the pelvic or abdominal peritoneum, where it can form new tumor nodules covering the lining of the pelvis or the lining of the abdomen or even replacing the omentum (the normal fatty structure that drapes between the stomach and transverse colon). This is a very common site in which to find advanced ovarian cancer. When the omentum is replaced with tumor, it is commonly described as an **omental cake**.

Another path for metastasis lies through the lymphatic channels. **Lymphatic channels** form a complex and extensive network of channels found throughout the body. They function to drain the body of waste. Ovarian carcinoma can spread through the lymph nodes of the pelvis into the periaortic area and occasionally can even spread to lymph nodes in the chest and neck region. Approximately 20% of apparent early ovarian cancer may have disease spread outside the ovary, particularly in lymph nodes. With advanced ovarian cancer, the lymph nodes may be involved in as many as 60% of patients.

Direct extension

The process by which cancer extends into local and surrounding tissue.

Omental cake

Tumor involvement of the omentum that results in the formation of a large mass.

Lymphatic channels

Vessels through which lymph fluid travels; part of the lymphatic system.

Metastasis can also take place through the bloodstream. When cancer invades into blood vessels, it can travel throughout the body, a process called **hematogenous dissemination**. It is through the bloodstream that ovarian cancer spreads to the lungs, liver, or brain.

Hematogenous dissemination

A process of spreading by which cancer travels through the bloodstream.

22. Should I get a second opinion? Could consulting another doctor affect my treatment or prognosis?

Choosing your doctor is ultimately a decision that can affect your outcome and your survival. Your primary physician probably handled matters through your initial diagnosis, and indeed may be a good person to assist you throughout your treatment. However, even if he or she is a gynecologist, your primary physician probably is not a specialist in treating ovarian cancer and therefore cannot be expected to be up to date on the latest information about this disease. Moreover, you are going to need surgery to remove the cancer, and that's something your primary physician cannot provide—but a **gynecologic oncologist** can. Thus, your outcome and chances of survival may be improved if you request from the beginning that a gynecologic oncologist be involved in your care, either as your primary surgeon or as a standby assistant surgeon. If you're diagnosed with ovarian cancer by your primary physician, please seek consultation with a gynecologic oncologist as soon as possible.

Gynecological oncologist

A specialist in the treatment of cancer of the female reproductive system.

You could also request a referral to a gynecologic oncologist to obtain a second opinion if you wish to be absolutely certain about the nature of your illness or the type of cancer and its treatment options.

A second opinion is always reasonable. In general, a second opinion is a good idea if surgery has been recommended, because the type and extent of the surgical procedure can affect overall treatment recommendations and may even alter your prognosis. Women who have all their cancer removed (complete resection) or have all but less than 1 centimeter of disease removed (optimal debulking) tend to fare better than do women whose cancer cannot be removed for technical reasons (suboptimal debulking). In general, a qualified gynecological oncologist, not a general surgeon or gynecologist, should perform any surgery for ovarian cancer.

When it comes to chemotherapy, a second opinion is reasonable, especially if you are uncertain about what treatment to take, if you are interested in a clinical trial (discussed in Question 42 on page 64), or if you are interested in a more aggressive approach beyond what is done routinely. Ongoing research is trying to improve on the results of standard treatment, and you should explore such research if you are interested. If a cancer comes back (recurs), a second opinion is very reasonable in order to explore clinical trials and the different ways to treat recurrent disease.

Dee's comment:

My gynecologist knew of the importance of having surgery done by a gynecologic oncologist if cancer was a possibility. I am glad that she referred me to Dr. Rodriguez, a gynecologic oncologist.

My situation is a bit unique, as there are a number of physicians in my family. I was able to turn to them for advice, as well as my primary care physician, whom I have seen for over 15 years. I was also able to reach out to my sister's oncologist for advice. They all concurred with my gynecologic oncologist's treatment plan so I felt comfortable with my decision to have her treat me.

I live in an area where there are multiple cancer centers within a 2-hour drive, so most women I know through support groups and awareness activities have received a second opinion at one of those centers. Many have also traveled to other institutions such as the NIH for consults about clinical trials.

My gynecologic oncologists have told me that if I wanted to investigate other treatment options that my records could easily be sent to physicians at other cancer centers. I believe most oncologists feel the same way, so you should not feel uncomfortable or think your doctor will be angry if you ask for your records to be sent to another doctor for a second opinion.

PART THREE

Treatment of Ovarian Cancer

How do I decide on where to be treated?

Who's involved in my treatment?

Who should do my surgery?

More...

23. How do I decide where to be treated?

Deciding where to obtain treatment is a very personal issue, and your comfort with your treating physician should guide you. Your relationship with your oncologist is going to be one of the most important relationships you have; for that reason, it must be based on trust and honesty. If you do not feel comfortable asking questions or you feel that your oncologist is not taking you seriously, you should find a new provider. Just as important is that your oncologist be accessible.

Surgery and medical treatments can result in side effects and complications that can require frequent visits to your doctor's office or may require you to go into a hospital. The distance you have to travel should also be a factor to consider. The worst situation is to feel sick but helpless because you live too far away.

24. Who's involved in my treatment?

It's important for you to be treated by a gynecologic oncologist because they are trained to specifically care for women with ovarian cancer. While all gynecologic oncologists are trained in all aspects of care (including medical treatment), not all gynecologic oncologists administer chemotherapy. Therefore, it is important that you be aware of the approach to treatment locally.

In specialized cancer centers, a gynecologic oncologist works with a medical oncologist who has a special interest and experience in the treatment of women with ovarian cancer. In addition, they may work with a radiation oncologist, who might be helpful to you in the future, if the disease were to recur.

Dee's comment:

Since I am treated at a comprehensive cancer center, I have access to a treatment team, which includes my gynecologic oncologists, advance practice nurses, oncology nurses, social workers, a dietitian, and pharmacists with special certifications in oncology. It took me a while to realize there were so many people on my team to whom I could look for support and information.

More than once, I consulted the pharmacist at my cancer center to discuss how best to take my medications when I was at home. I was taking medications for other conditions too, and he was able to tell me the best time to take them so they would not interact with my nausea and pain medications. We also discussed the use of over-the-counter drugs and vitamins.

During treatment, I frequently made calls to the nurse help line at Rutgers Cancer Institute of New Jersey. Some of the questions I asked them were about some pain I was having, what to avoid when I was neutropenic, and what to take for gas.

Other members of the treatment team are the pathologist, nurses, and even advanced practice providers (like nurse practitioners and physician assistants). In addition to these clinicians, it is important to have access to the supporting staff in the office, including but not limited to the social workers and clinical therapists who can help you and your loved ones adjust to often difficult situations.

SURGERY

25. Who should do my surgery?

If a diagnosis of ovarian cancer is suspected or if the possibility of ovarian cancer is present, surgery should be performed by a gynecologic oncologist. Gynecologic oncologists are physicians who have completed a full training in general obstetrics and gynecology and have received additional specialized training in gynecologic oncology (usually 2–4 years).

Surgery for ovarian cancer is best performed where the appropriate operation can be conducted and resection of advanced disease can be as complete as possible. Unfortunately, many patients with ovarian cancer continue to have their surgery performed by non-oncologic surgeons; this results in an incomplete operation or a less aggressive attempt at resection. In such situations, a patient may require additional surgery in order to stage the disease completely or to resect advanced disease.

26. What will the surgeon do?

The first things that the surgeon will do are study your medical history; perform a thorough examination, including a pelvic examination; and review any radiology studies. If the history review and examination suggest ovarian cancer, your surgeon will recommend surgery. The goals of surgery are to remove the primary cancer, to determine whether the cancer has spread, and to attempt to remove the spread of cancer as best as possible.

SURGERY FOR APPARENTLY EARLY DISEASE

If radiology exams indicate that you have localized or early ovarian cancer (generally meaning the disease is contained only within your pelvis), the surgeon will remove both your fallopian tubes and ovaries and your uterus. That's described as a total abdominal hysterectomy and bilateral salpingo-oophorectomy. In addition, your surgeon will take samples from any areas of possible tumor spread as part of the staging procedure.

That would mean taking the lymph nodes from both sides of your pelvis and around the aorta, removal of the omentum, and obtaining tissue from around your abdomen and pelvis (known as peritoneal biopsies) and washings to exclude cancer spread. If disease is present in your abdomen at the time of surgery, the goal of surgery would be to debulk or resect as much as possible, leaving the smallest possible amount of visible disease.

ADVANCED DISEASE

When ovarian cancer is advanced or widespread, more extensive surgery is usually needed, and you would likely undergo radical debulking. It is important to know that the description that follows applies only to selected patients with advanced bulky disease; it is not what early-stage ovarian cancer patients undergo. However, it provides ample reason for a newly diagnosed patient to avoid delaying treatment.

Debulking usually requires a resection of the uterus, both tubes and ovaries, possibly the rectum, and part of the large colon. If that were the case, you might require a segment of bowel pulled through your abdomen so that stool can drain (a **colostomy**). This intestinal diversion is usually temporary and may be reversed by another operation at a later date.

Colostomy

A loop of bowel that is pulled through your skin.

Occasionally, segments of small intestine have to be removed. The lining of the abdomen may have implants on it, and these are also removed. Occasionally, the lining of the diaphragm also will have to be removed.

Less frequently, patients may have advanced disease involving their liver or gallbladder; in such cases, resection of these areas may become necessary. The spleen is another organ that occasionally can be involved in ovarian cancer. It is not uncommon for women to undergo a splenectomy in order to remove disease that may be involving the spleen. Occasionally, the appendix is removed as part of ovarian cancer surgery. The overall intent is to completely remove all visible sites of disease, sometimes referred to as debulking to no gross residual disease or a complete cytoreduction.

If a surgeon finds the disease is too advanced and cannot be completely removed, or a woman's overall health makes surgery highly risky, then primary treatment may consist of chemotherapy, sometimes called **neoadjuvant treatment**. This approach aims to decrease the volume of cancer with medical therapy (typically three cycles of chemotherapy) before you undergo an operation (called an interval debulking). A large clinical trial of women compared those who had an initial attempt at debulking and then were randomized to chemotherapy versus those who had chemotherapy for three cycles followed by surgery and more chemotherapy afterwards; no survival advantage was seen with interval surgery. Still, it was not any less successful, either.

Neoadjuvant treatment

Treatment given before surgery.

27. Must the surgeon remove both ovaries if I am diagnosed with ovarian cancer?

Most ovarian cancer patients are postmenopausal, so concerns about fertility are irrelevant in the majority of cases. Some patients, however, are diagnosed before menopause, and a certain proportion of young women are concerned about maintaining their ability to have children in the future. If you have completed your family and have no desire to remain fertile, the standard of care is to remove both your ovaries and fallopian tubes and your uterus and to perform a staging operation. This has been the

TREATMENT OF OVARIAN CANCER

traditional surgical method of treating ovarian cancer, and it is the most likely method to prevent future recurrence. However, if you strongly desire to preserve your ability to have children and have no obvious spread of cancer outside your ovary, it may possible to retain your uterus and the uninvolved tube but proceed with a full staging operation. In that procedure, the uterus and the uninvolved tube and ovary are left intact and are not removed, which would allow a woman to have children in the future. Yet even in the case of fertility-sparing surgery, the operation should still include a complete staging, which would include removal of the lymph nodes and the omentum and obtaining the peritoneal biopsies. It is not clear what risks a woman takes when she undergoes conservative surgery to preserve her chances of having or carrying a baby later. Results presented from the Memorial Sloan-Kettering Cancer show that selected women undergoing conservative surgery had similar long-term survival compared to women undergoing complete surgical treatment. However, the number of women studied was small and the subject requires further studies.

28. What if I wasn't staged—should I go back to the operating room?

Surgical staging is extremely important if you are diagnosed with ovarian cancer. Staging is usually performed by an operation via an incision in the abdomen or sometimes by **laparoscopy**. Staging requires the evaluation of the pelvic and abdominal organs in the peritoneal cavity and retroperitoneum with multiple biopsies, washings, removal of lymph nodes, sampling of any suspicious areas in the abdomen, and removal of the omentum. Staging also requires that an evaluation of the chest with a chest x-ray or a CT scan be performed to ensure that the lungs are free of disease. If your cancer appears

Laparoscopy

Camera-directed surgery done without creating a large incision in the abdomen.

to be limited to the ovary (stage I disease), surgical staging gains more importance. Anywhere between 20% and 30% of women who appear to have disease limited to the ovary will be found to have microscopic or small-volume disease outside the ovary when staged. This may profoundly affect their postsurgical treatment, particularly regarding chemotherapy options.

Today, many centers will treat advanced stage III ovarian carcinoma that has been successfully removed (also known as an optimal cytoreduction) with a combination of intravenous and intraperitoneal chemotherapy. If an adequate staging is not performed, it will be unlikely that patients with stage III disease based on microscopic disease will be identified. If you have been diagnosed with ovarian cancer and were not staged at that time, the decision of whether you should go back for a second surgery will depend on what was found at that first operation. If the disease appeared to be extensive and the patient will need prompt initiation of systemic chemotherapy, it may not be absolutely necessary to return for restaging. Still, staging should be considered in all women diagnosed with ovarian cancer.

29. What is an intravenous MediPort? Should I get one?

A MediPort is a device made up of a small elastic tube connected to a **reservoir** that can be placed in the body under local anesthesia. It allows us to give medications and chemotherapy intravenously. The reservoir is usually placed over the rib cage and below the right or left collar bone, or alternatively, it can be placed in the arm. These catheters or reservoirs can then be removed in the clinic when chemotherapy is completed, usually under local anesthesia, without much difficulty.

Reservoir

A receptacle that holds fluid.

The catheters are introduced through a large vein deep in the chest and the reservoir is fixed to the chest wall under the skin. These MediPorts allow administration of intravenous fluids, medications, and chemotherapy and also allow for drawing of blood periodically. The advantage of the MediPort is that it will avoid multiple peripheral phlebotomy and venous sticks in the arms, and the central MediPort can be used for the majority of intravenous blood draws or administration of medication. These ports are usually placed by an interventional radiologist under local anesthesia or by a gynecologic oncologist or a surgeon in the operating room. The ports can be removed under local anesthesia, either bedside or in the outpatient office setting. If you have a difficult vein to access and you have a hard time having blood drawn or starting intravenous infusion, insertion of a venous MediPort may be a good option. This MediPort can be removed at the end of chemotherapy.

Dee's comment:

I had IV chemotherapy, although now both IV and IP may be used to administer chemotherapy drugs. My veins were hard to access, so my gynecologic oncologist recommended a chest port-a-catheter (a central MediPort) for IV chemotherapy. I am very happy I agreed to the minor surgery involved to insert the port.

I had my port inserted in the hospital's interventional radiology department in a relatively quick, same-day surgery. My chest was uncomfortable for a few days after the surgery, but it was worth it to not be poked multiple times to insert the IV.

If you have a port be sure to ask your doctor for some numbing (lidocaine) cream. I would start putting the cream on the skin over my port about an hour before it was to be accessed. When it was accessed I felt some pressure but no pain at all.

TREATMENT OF OVARIAN CANCER

If you keep your port after treatment is finished, be sure you have it flushed on a regular basis. I had mine for 9 years. I would get it flushed regularly (every 4–8 weeks), and never had issue with its functionality.

MEDICAL THERAPY

30. Does everyone with ovarian cancer need medical therapy?

Medical therapy most often means chemotherapy, but it also includes other newer forms of treatment, such as drugs that inhibit blood vessel formation (i.e., **angiogenesis inhibitors**), antihormonal treatment (or endocrine therapy), and even a newer class of drugs called **poly-ADP ribose polymerase (PARP) inhibitors**, which are indicated for women with recurrent ovarian cancer associated with a BRCA gene mutation.

In general, chemotherapy is recommended for every patient with ovarian cancer except those with stage IA, grade 1 or grade 2 tumors. Grade 3 cancers, even at the earliest stages, are usually treated with chemotherapy. Two large trials in women with early-stage disease suggested that the addition of chemotherapy to surgery improves overall survival by 8% and improves the chances of not having it come back by 11%, compared to surgery alone.

31. What kind of agents are used to treat newly diagnosed ovarian cancer?

Landmark clinical trials have established that standard treatment of newly diagnosed epithelial ovarian cancer uses a taxane-platinum combination. In addition, the

Angiogenesis inhibitors

Drugs that block the formation of new blood vessels.

Poly-ADP ribose polymerase (PARP) inhibitors

They block proteins involved in the repair of DNA breaks.

angiogenesis inhibitor, bevacizumab, may be used in the adjuvant (or first-line) setting. These drugs are described below. Other drugs used to treat recurrent ovarian cancer are addressed in Question 77 on page 108 and listed in **Table 5**.

Platinum agents (carboplatin and cisplatin) are the drugs most active in treating ovarian cancer; they work by creating breaks in the DNA, leading eventually to cell death. They can be given either by vein or directly into the abdomen (**intraperitoneal** treatment). Although active against cancer cells, they also affect normally dividing cells, which accounts for some of their side effects (discussed later).

Intraperitoneal
Into the abdomen.

Taxanes (paclitaxel, docetaxel) work by blocking microtubules (tiny structures important in the process of cells dividing). Paclitaxel was the drug initially studied in clinical trials involving ovarian cancer patients. It is given over 24 hours, if combined with cisplatin, or as a 3-hour infusion when given with carboplatin, which is the more common chemotherapy program used. Recently, a large European study confirmed that docetaxel is equivalent to paclitaxel, but has fewer long-term side effects than paclitaxel.

Angiogenesis inhibitors appear to be very active in ovarian cancer, and among the best studied is bevacizumab. Two trials showed that using bevacizumab as part of an initial treatment strategy increases the time that a woman is free of cancer, but ultimately, there was no evidence that it improved overall survival. However, in one of these studies, women at the highest risk of recurrence appeared to benefit from adjuvant bevacizumab.

32. How is medical treatment administered?

This depends on the outcome of surgery and the practice pattern at your hospital. At specialized centers, the outcomes of surgery is often used to determine the best treatment.

Intravenous (IV) Plus Intraperitoneal (IP) administration. For women with stage II or stage III disease and for whom the gynecologic oncologist successfully removed all or most of your disease (optimal debulking), a combination of intravenous (IV) and intraperitoneal (IP) treatment may be used. A common schedule is to give paclitaxel IV on day one, cisplatin IP on day 2, and then paclitaxel IP on day 8, with treatment repeated every 21 days for up to six cycles. This schedule was shown to result in the longest overall survival reported on a randomized trial. However, this regimen is more complicated than intravenous treatment alone, and may require a hospital stay to get the treatment.

The IP route requires placement of a temporary catheter in your abdomen that's connected to a small plastic container (a reservoir) positioned underneath the skin, usually right on top of your lower rib cage (**Figures 4** and **5**). The reservoir can be accessed with a needle through the skin, which allows drugs to be given directly into your abdomen. The agents are allowed to spread throughout the peritoneal cavity (hence the term **belly wash**) and eventually are absorbed through the abdominal lining over the next 1 to 2 days. This method of administering chemotherapy is attractive for patients with ovarian cancer because this disease tends to spread through the lining of the abdomen and, in many cases, stays in the peritoneal cavity.

Belly wash

Common term for an intraperitoneal treatment.

The IP catheter and reservoir are removed after the treatment is completed. This generally does not require a large surgery and is often performed in an outpatient setting under local anesthesia without much difficulty or complications. The IP catheter and reservoir, like any other foreign device in humans, carry a small risk of infection or malfunction, and occasionally the catheter has to be removed due to either malfunction or infection.

The main side effects during the treatment are feeling distended or cramping during administration of

IP Catheter

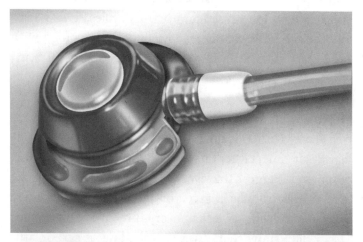

Figure 4
IP catheter
and reservoir
(BardPort type).

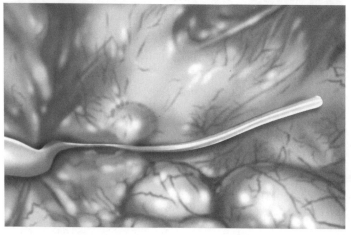

Figure 5
IP catheter placed
in the pelvis.

the chemotherapeutic agent. However, the drug can be absorbed into your bloodstream, and this can cause side effects.

IV treatment. For women with early-stage ovarian cancer and those with advanced disease who are not candidates for IP treatment, including those who refuse IP treatment for whatever reason, IV chemotherapy is indicated. However, treatment can be administered on several schedules.

The most common administration schedule is to give both carboplatin and paclitaxel on the same day (day 1) every 21 days (one cycle) for up to six cycles. This is usually the schedule that is recommended for women with early-stage disease and is reasonable for all other women who are not going to receive IP chemotherapy.

However, treatment can also be administered more frequently (called a dose-dense schedule). On a dose-dense schedule, either one or both drugs is given weekly. Some data suggest that weekly administration of paclitaxel with carboplatin given on day 1 only (of a 21-day cycle) is more effective than every three week treatment. Other data show that a weekly schedule of carboplatin plus paclitaxel is as good as every three week treatment, and may be better tolerated. Such an option might be reasonable for older or more frail patients who are still candidates for chemotherapy.

While there is no consensus on whether or not to use bevacizumab in the first-line setting, for some patients and their doctors, a chance to prolong the time that ovarian cancer does not grow (or the progression-free survival interval) may be sufficient justification to proceed with treatment. If administered, bevacizumab is usually given every three weeks during chemotherapy and then continued for up to one year total duration (sometimes called maintenance treatment). At least some data suggest that using bevacizumab may be more important in women at greater risk of having a recurrence, including those with stage IV (or metastatic) ovarian cancer and those with stage III disease who had > 1 cm residual disease after surgery (or were suboptimally resected).

33. What are the side effects of chemotherapy? What about bevacizumab? What about other agents?

Platinum agents. Cisplatin has significant side effects, including nausea and vomiting, potential hearing loss, kidney injury, and permanent nerve damage. Fortunately, we have learned through clinical trials that a very close cousin to cisplatin—carboplatin—is just as effective. Carboplatin is also less likely to injure the kidneys and nerves. Its major toxicity lies in decreasing your blood counts, which can make you prone to infection.

Taxanes. The major side effects of paclitaxel are total hair loss, with the most dramatic loss occurring after the first treatment, as well as numbness, tingling, or both, usually affecting the hands and feet. That sensation is usually reversible after paclitaxel is stopped. In addition, paclitaxel can cause a hypersensitivity reaction (your body reacting to what it thinks is a foreign substance) while the drug is being infused into your system. The reaction usually occurs during the start of the infusion and can occur during any of your treatments. It can be characterized by many types of symptoms: flushing, shortness of breath, chest pressure, chest or back pain, or rash. It can usually be managed by stopping the infusion and giving

Antihistamine

To block the release of histamines, which are often associated with allergic reactions.

Cremaphore

A molecule to which drugs are attached to increase the drugs' delivery into your body.

you an extra dose of **antihistamines**. Once the reaction subsides, paclitaxel can be restarted. This is because the reaction is caused not by paclitaxel itself but by the molecule with which it is mixed to allow it to be absorbed better into your bloodstream. Your body may react to this other substance (called a **cremaphore**) by releasing histamines that cause the reaction. Once your body releases all its histamines, the infusion can be restarted. In order to decrease the risk of hypersensitivity reactions, premedication with steroids (usually dexamethasone) is used prior to treatment, starting the night before you get paclitaxel.

Docetaxel does not cause the same degree of numbness or tingling, although it does cause hair loss. Its major side effect is decreased blood counts, which can be treated with medications that boost blood cell production. Other side effects of docetaxel are hypersensitivity reactions and fluid build-up, which can cause your face, arms, or legs to swell. The risk for both of these side effects can be reduced with the use of steroid premedication.

Fatigue or tiredness is a common effect of treatment that can get worse as you approach the end of your treatment (i.e., the fifth and sixth treatments). This may last for a couple of months, but then you should slowly start to feel like yourself once it is completed.

Other chemotherapy agents. Most other chemotherapy drugs have similar side effects, including effects on the bone marrow, causing anemia, low platelets, or lowering white cells (and making you at risk of infections). Some of the drugs commonly used to treat ovarian cancer, however, do have drug-specific side effects. Liposomal doxorubicin can cause a red, scaling, and sometimes painful rash that can affect the hands and feet, and is called a hand-foot syndrome. Gemcitabine can cause low-grade fevers the day after it is given or even difficulty breathing or pleural effusions. Etoposide and hexamethylamine are oral agents that cause nausea and vomiting as their major toxicity. Topotecan can cause nausea as well, but its major toxicity is on the bone marrow. Table 5 in Question 77 outlines the drugs that are routinely used to treat ovarian cancer and summarizes the major side effects of treatment.

Bevacizumab. Bevacizumab causes side effects that are not like the usual effects of chemotherapy. It can increase the blood pressure to the point that medication (sometimes multiple drugs) are required to control it. It can also cause bleeding, delayed wound healing, and problems with the kidney, including spilling protein in the urine (**proteinuria**). There is a risk for a bowel perforation as well, though it appears to happen in only 2–3% of cases. In addition, we think that some clinical features increase the risk of a **bowel perforation**, such as multiple prior treatments for cancer and a recent history of bowel dysfunction, including bowel obstruction.

Olaparib. Olaparib is an orally administered, targeted therapy drug that blocks the activity of a protein called poly-ADP ribose polymerase (PARP); hence, it is called a PARP inhibitor. It is thought that certain cancer cells rely on PARP to help them repair their DNA, thus keeping the cells alive and allowing them to divide and grow. Medications that inhibit PARP are therefore thought to decrease the opportunities for these specific cancer cells to grow. Olaparib was approved in the US specifically for women with recurrent ovarian cancer associated with a BRCA1 or BRCA2 genetic mutation following disease progression after at least three different treatments of chemotherapy. The most common side effects are gastrointestinal, including nausea and vomiting, and

Proteinuria

The spilling of protein by the kidneys, which is picked up by a urine evaluation.

Bowel perforation

A rupture of the bowel wall.

Dyspepsia

Pain in the stomach.

Myelodysplastic syndrome

Abnormal development of blood cells that represents a problem in the bone marrow.

dyspepsia. It can also cause weakness or fatigue and musculoskeletal pain. Although not well characterized, there may be risk for a more serious hematologic disorder called **myelodysplastic syndrome** or even acute myelogenous leukemia and for lung inflammation (known as pneumonitis). Researchers are still trying to quantify the risk to patients for this particular side effect.

Additional information from AstraZeneca is provided as follows.

Olaparib. Olaparib (tradename LYNPARZA) is an oral poly-ADP ribose polymerase (PARP) inhibitor and is a medicine available by prescription to treat women with advanced ovarian cancer who have received previous treatment with 3 or more prior chemotherapy medicines or a combination of chemotherapy medicines for their cancer, and have a certain type of abnormal inherited BRCA gene. A healthcare provider will perform a test to make sure that olaparib is right for the patient. The most important information one should know about olaparib is that it may cause serious side effects that can lead to death, including: Bone marrow problems called Myelodysplastic Syndrome (MDS) or Acute Myeloid Leukemia (AML) and Lung problems (pneumonitis). Healthcare providers will perform blood tests to check a patients' blood cell counts before treatment, every month during treatment, and also weekly if one has low blood cell counts that last a long time. Treatment may be stopped until blood cell counts improve. Olaparib may cause serious side effects. The most common include: nausea or vomiting, tiredness or weakness, diarrhea, indigestion or heartburn, headache, loss of appetite, changes in the way food tastes, changes in kidney function blood tests, sore throat or runny nose, upper respiratory infection, cough, pain in the joints, muscles, and back, rash, and pain or discomfort in the stomach area. These are not all the possible side effects of olaparib. **See accompanying Full Prescribing Information, including Patient Information (Medication Guide) for complete risk information, or visit www.lynparza.com.**

TREATMENT OF NONEPITHELIAL OVARIAN CANCER

34. When do germ-cell tumors require chemotherapy?

In women diagnosed with early-stage disease, postsurgical treatment using chemotherapy is usually reserved for those with any of the following types of tumors: embryonal carcinomas, endodermal sinus tumors, or mixed germ-cell tumors. Women with these types of tumors are at a high risk of relapse, so chemotherapy is given after surgery in the hope that the drugs will destroy any tumor cells that might remain after surgery and thus prevent recurrence. Chemotherapy is also given in women who have advanced germ-cell tumors or in whom tumors have returned.

The general treatment uses drugs different from those used for epithelial cancers. The most common regimen (program or schedule) is bleomycin, etoposide, and cisplatin (BEP). It has been shown to be very active in the treatment of germ-cell cancers. However, this regimen is not without risks, and the potential benefit of treatment has to be weighed against the side effects of the treatment. Because women with germ-cell tumors are typically young when they are diagnosed, these considerations should not be taken lightly.

The major side effects that need to be considered are damage from bleomycin to your lungs, which can happen during or after treatment and can lead to scarring (or **pulmonary fibrosis**); damage from cisplatin to your nerves and kidneys, which can be permanent; and a risk (although rare) from etoposide of causing leukemia later in life.

Pulmonary fibrosis

Scarring of the lung tissue, which may or may not be reversible.

More than 90% of patients with germ-cell tumors will be cured after the BEP program. The number of treatments is generally three or four cycles given every 3 weeks, although your physician may recommend more if your disease has spread or if treatment has to be changed due to side effects that occur while you're on BEP.

35. Do all types of sex cord–stromal tumors require chemotherapy?

No, not all sex cord or stromal tumors require chemotherapy. Many of these tumors will require only surgery, but it's important that surgical staging be complete, particularly in women who want to keep their fertility.

Early-stage granulosa-cell tumors do not warrant treatment after surgery. Even for women with advanced disease, the benefit of postoperative treatment with radiation, chemotherapy, or hormones is not completely clear. In such a case, your oncologist may recommend no further treatment except regular visits to the office every 3 to 4 months.

Even when disease recurs, surgery is the preferred choice of treatment. Your oncologist may offer chemotherapy, but this decision is an individual choice based on how much cancer was found, the length of time before the cancer came back, and how strong you are at the time of the recurrence. If chemotherapy becomes necessary, the regimen of choice is BEP. The optimal management for women with recurrent or incompletely resected disease has not been established.

36. Is chemotherapy ever recommended for borderline tumors?

Chemotherapy has no standard role in treating borderline tumors. The major treatment is surgical. If the entire tumor is removed, particularly if it is found at an early stage, women with these tumors are generally cured. Even if the disease has spread outside your pelvis, all attempts at removing all visible disease afford the best chance of survival; chemotherapy may or may not be recommended. In general, chemotherapy is reserved for tumors that were incompletely removed surgically or else are found through the microscope to be invasive (which can signify a more aggressive tendency to the borderline tumor, or even actual cancer). If chemotherapy is warranted, the tumor is treated with carboplatin and paclitaxel, just as for ovarian cancer.

37. Are any tumor markers associated with these nonepithelial types of ovarian tumors?

CA-125 results are sometimes increased in women with borderline tumors.

For the germ-cell tumors, two types of proteins are often elevated. These are the human chorionic gonadotropin (or the hCG) and alpha-fetoprotein (AFP). The hCG is what is tested in a pregnancy test, but in this situation it is used to monitor the activity of both nongestational choriocarcinomas and dysgerminomas during treatment. AFP is a tumor marker as well, and is elevated in endodermal sinus tumors, immature teratoma, and the embryonal carcinomas.

The sex cord–stromal tumors can cause increased estrogen and progesterone levels but do not usually have a tumor marker. One exception is the granulosa-cell tumor, which secretes a protein known as inhibin. Other useful markers may include LDH and CA-125.

MONITORING DURING TREATMENT

38. How will I be monitored during treatment?

It is important that you have an exam prior to the start of each new cycle, sometimes called "pre-treatment clearance". A provider should meet with you to see how the prior treatment and subsequent weeks went for you, so that they can help address any side effects you may have experienced. Since some drugs can cause side effects that might last well beyond the completion of treatment (like neuropathy), it is important to identify them as early as possible. If side effects appear to be an issue, your provider might delay treatment until you feel better or may even reduce the dose (or doses) of the agents being used to treat your cancer.

In addition, during these visits, your provider will re-evaluate your progress. For women with ovarian cancer, they do this by repeating a pelvic exam to make sure there is nothing suspicious that can be felt within the vaginal vault, a review of your basic bloodwork (to check for anemia, kidney function, and your liver's status), and your CA-125, if it was elevated at the time you were first diagnosed. In addition to CA-125, your doctors may order monitoring using another blood test for a human epididymis protein, called HE4. It may be particularly useful if the CA-125 is not elevated.

39. What happens if the CA-125 result isn't normal during chemotherapy?

The CA-125 reading should decrease gradually with treatment. Ideally, it should be normal after the third treatment, although this may depend on how high the CA-125 result was when you started treatment. If it is going down slowly, your doctor may recommend additional cycles of treatment, usually up to eight cycles. If the number flattens out or starts to rise, it may indicate that your cancer is not responding to the treatment. It is important that a repeat evaluation be performed in that situation, usually with a CT scan. Signs signaling that the disease isn't responding call for a change in plan, because more of the same treatment is unlikely to help you.

If your disease stops responding to up-front treatment, your doctor may describe your cancer as "primary platinum-refractory." In women with platinum-refractory disease, the cancer is not curable. Instead, the goal of further therapy becomes one of control. This approach is similar to that taken for women with recurrent ovarian cancer, particularly if the cancer comes back in a short time (within 3 months of stopping treatment). The management (handling) of recurrent and refractory cancers is discussed later in this book (see **Part Six**).

40. Does radiation play a role in treatment?

Although it's not considered a standard treatment for ovarian cancer, radiation is an effective means of treatment. It has fallen out of favor as **adjuvant** treatment (i.e., after surgery) because chemotherapy has been shown to be an effective means of therapy. When used after initial surgery, radiation is directed against the entire abdomen; this carries a risk of complications to your bowel and kidneys. Therefore, it's usually reserved for treatment of recurrent tumors, particularly in situations in which an isolated recurrence can be encompassed in one radiation field.

Adjuvant

Given after a primary procedure.

41. What is the role of immunotherapy in ovarian cancer?

We believe that the immune system is important in how the body fights ovarian cancer. Some studies show that the presence of immune cells within the tumor predicts a better outcome. How to harness the power of the immune system is an important area of clinical research. One example is the studies on cancer vaccines. **Vaccines** are a novel way to try to stop cancer by teaching the body's immune system to recognize tumor cells as foreign and kill them off. Some vaccines are individualized, based on one's own tumor, while others are based on the common molecules found on the majority of ovarian cancers, such as the cancer protein, CA-125. To date, immunotherapy is investigational. However, it is a very promising area of research and anyone interested should look for clinical trials they can participate in.

Vaccine

A preparation that is given to induce immunity to a disease or condition.

42. When should I consider a clinical trial?

Participating in clinical trials (studies using patients) is always an option for women in all phases of ovarian cancer, from initial diagnosis to relapse to second remission. However, the vast majority of women turn to clinical trials only after standard therapy has failed.

There are no guidelines in place as to when a patient should participate in a clinical trial. Before you begin investigating trial options, it is important to understand the different types of studies done in cancer research, because not all trials are the same, and you need to look for one that is suited to your circumstances.

There are three basic types of clinical trials. Phase I trials are the earliest type of clinical trials. They are designed to test a new medication or treatment strategy, and often they are "first-in-human" studies involving only a small number of patients. The main purpose of these trials is to determine the best dose of a new drug or treatment to take into further development. This is done by starting at a low dose and gradually increasing it until side effects are seen. This leads us to the second goal of these early trials: to determine what kind of side effects are associated with the new treatment being tested. It's important to realize that although most phase I trials want to test whether the study drug can cause tumors to shrink, it is not the primary goal.

Once a phase I trial is completed, the next step in development of a new treatment is to define how active a drug is. That's the goal of a phase II trial. Unlike phase I trials, the majority of phase II trials are conducted to target specific diseases. In general, all patients enrolled in these studies are treated with the study medication.

The vast majority of women turn to clinical trials only after standard therapy has failed.

TREATMENT OF OVARIAN CANCER

If a drug or treatment looks promising in a phase II trial, the next step—a phase III trial—involves comparing it against an accepted treatment in a specific disease setting. The goal is to determine whether the treatment being tested is better than the current available treatment. These are usually run as randomized trials (participating patients are assigned randomly to a treatment). Neither they nor their doctors can select the treatment they'll receive. The results of these trials usually determine the standard of care for oncologists.

For women with newly diagnosed ovarian cancer, phase II and phase III trials are available nationally, either through research centers as single-institution studies (meaning that a certain type of treatment is being studied in only one place) or as part of a cooperative group trial (meaning that patients are being offered the trial in multiple places). For women with recurrent cancers of the ovary, both types of trials may be available. Many of the trials limit entry by the number of prior therapies, which are decided by the physicians and scientists studying the treatment.

Often, patients who have had two or three different treatments are excluded from the trial; although exclusion is a controversial subject (no one wants to be denied a treatment that could save her life), there are some legitimate concerns that cause investigators to refuse women previously treated with other medications access to the trial. For example, many chemotherapy regimens are toxic, not just to cancer cells, but to organs such as the liver or the kidneys. If the clinical trial drug is thought to be equally or more toxic, the investigators might be concerned that women with toxicity from prior therapy could get sicker, not healthier, by participating in the trial. Fortunately, these concerns are less significant in trials of the new targeted therapies, so women previously treated with other drugs can often be admitted into such trials. Nevertheless, this consideration is important because it may affect your options to receive standard treatments before you enter the study.

It's important to understand that the purpose of a clinical trial is to test a theory, in this case usually a question regarding the effectiveness of a new treatment strategy. If something is being tested in a clinical trial, its benefit is still unproven. It's never wrong to explore clinical trial options for any stage of ovarian cancer, however, and remember: All of the current standard therapies were once unproven—they only became standard therapies because they passed through clinical trials. However, the goals of the trial should be clearly stated and understood before you make the decision. (See the **Additional Resources** for more information on clinical trials.)

Dee's comment:

I was offered a clinical trial when I was first diagnosed. It was a phase I trial that included selenium along with the standard drugs (carboplatin and paclitaxel). The selenium was being added to help with the chemoresistance that some women develop when treated with carboplatin. It was explained to me that the trial was testing the dosage levels and side effects of the addition of the selenium. I also knew that I would not necessarily gain any benefit due to its addition.

After telling my gynecologic oncologist that I would consider the trial, I began by researching the drug with the help of the librarian at my cancer center. I read journal articles on initial tests with mice, as well as trials that used selenium to treat other cancers. Then I asked questions, lots and lots of questions, of the clinical trial nurse. There were other things I had to consider too when making my decision, such as the extra days at the cancer center for the selenium infusion and longer hours in the treatment area for additional blood work. After discussing it with my family, who would be impacted by the extra days at the cancer center, I decided to take part in the trial.

When I recurred I was much more comfortable considering a clinical trial right up front, since I had such a good experience the first time around. There was a perfect trial for recurrent ovarian cancer patients, but it required that I be randomized to surgery first or chemotherapy first. Since I felt strongly about having the surgery first, I declined the trial and had surgery.

I hope that as more women learn about clinical trials they will consider them not as a final step but earlier in their treatment plan. I know I will consider another clinical trial if I should recur.

43. Does treatment differ if I'm pregnant when diagnosed with ovarian cancer?

Most women who get ovarian cancer do so after menopause. Pregnancy-associated ovarian cancer is a rare, but devastating, diagnosis. It can occur in 1 in 12,000 to 50,000 pregnancies. Often the diagnosis is made surgically, after women present with an abnormal routine ultrasound showing a complex cyst. CT scans are not safe during pregnancy; however, if a complex cyst is found by ultrasound in a pregnant patient, then an MRI may be done.

The first step in management is surgical, as it would be if you were not pregnant. Every attempt should be made at complete surgical staging, which means that an open procedure or laparotomy must be performed.

Unfortunately, the decisions are not ones made easily. If you have advanced cancer with spread around the pelvis or abdomen, then your doctors may recommend that the pregnancy be terminated so that the most aggressive treatment can be used to give you the best chance of surviving the cancer. If you are early-staged but considered at a high risk for recurrence, some may advocate delaying treatment until after the first trimester, or even after the birth of your child, whereas others may recommend a more aggressive course. On the other end of the spectrum, you may be considered cured after the affected ovary is removed.

If, whatever the circumstance, you decide to continue with the pregnancy, your doctors must take into account your life first and foremost, all the while minimizing the potential risk to the unborn child.

There's not much information to help guide the postsurgical treatment of ovarian cancer in pregnancy. What we do know is that chemotherapy isn't safe during the first trimester, when all of your baby's organs are forming. However, beyond that, it can be safely administered, although there's always the risk of side effects.

Of the chemotherapy available to treat ovarian cancer, the little data available suggest that cisplatin is safe during pregnancy. Carboplatin may also be used, although the risk for lowering of the platelets (thrombocytopenia) may make cisplatin the better choice. The data on paclitaxel is much less clear, and there are only limited data on its use in pregnant women. In women with early-stage disease, the potential benefits of chemotherapy must be weighed against the risks of treatment.

Numerous factors must be taken into account, and you, your family, your oncologist, and your obstetrician must

TREATMENT OF OVARIAN CANCER

engage in a thorough and honest discussion about the pros and cons of all your options.

44. Is there any role for complementary or alternative therapy?

Alternative therapy (medicines used in lieu of standard medical therapies) and complementary therapy (medicines used in conjunction with standard therapies) include a variety of herbal and food remedies, vitamins and other supplements, and traditional treatments such as acupuncture. Such therapies have become increasingly popular with the general public, and many are based upon traditional healing practices that have hundreds of years of use. Whether they actually work is difficult to know due to the lack of clinical trials available on these types of treatments.

Some alternative therapies are nothing more than scams taking advantage of patients' fears and longings for anything that will make the illness go away. They may do no harm—although some herbal agents can harm you—but they also do no good, so you're spending your money for no good reason. For example, there are data strongly suggesting that the use of antioxidants can actually be harmful during chemotherapy treatment.

Some alternative healing practices also address some of the emotional and physiological problems that accompany cancer treatment, so using them may improve the patient's quality of life, even if it doesn't necessarily stop the cancer itself.

Many people are becoming attracted to alternative philosophies of patient care, particularly east and south Asian methods and homeopathic and naturopathic medical systems. Yet there are so many medicines and therapies touted as the next new treatment for cancer, it's hard to know where to start. For a cancer patient anxious to find an effective treatment—or even a way to deal with unpleasant treatment side effects—the list can be bewildering. A recent study of cancer patients showed that as many of 80% were using or had tried such treatments in conjunction with their standard therapeutic regimens, in the hope of either enhancing the action of the regimen or reducing the side effects caused by it. Unfortunately, a large proportion of the patients in the study were taking these alternative therapies without letting their doctors know and suffering side effects as the therapies interfered with or interacted with the action of chemotherapy drugs—which is why many physicians are wary of alternative medicines. Yet part of the problem is that doctors fail to ask whether their patients are using alternative therapies, and patients don't think to tell them. So the most important point to make in any discussion of alternative therapies is: Make sure your doctor knows about them before you start using them.

Relaxation Therapy. Although there isn't much research on the topic of alternative medicine, it's safe to assume that therapy aimed at relaxing the mind can have a positive impact on a patient fighting cancer. Relaxation therapy, including massage, yoga, or tai chi, may provide a benefit to the patient by relieving the psychological stress associated with a cancer diagnosis.

Homeopathic and Naturopathic Medicine. Homeopathic and naturopathic medicines are also examples of complete alternative medical systems. Homeopathic medicine is an unconventional Western system that is based on the principle that "like cures like"; that is, that the same substance that in large doses produces the symptoms of an illness, in very minute doses cures it. Naturopathic medicine views disease as a sign that the processes by which the body naturally heals itself are out of balance and emphasizes health restoration rather than disease treatment. Naturopathic physicians employ an array of healing practices, including diet and clinical nutrition; homeopathy; acupuncture; herbal medicine; hydrotherapy (the use of water in a range of temperatures and methods of applications); spinal and soft-tissue manipulation; physical therapies involving electric currents, ultrasound, and light therapy; therapeutic counseling; and pharmacology. Regarding homeopathic and naturopathic remedies, some physicians may recommend not taking antioxidants while on chemotherapy. This is because, in theory, chemotherapy acts by causing oxidative damage to cancer cells, so antioxidants could work against the activity of chemotherapy. If you're going to use alternative medications while undergoing treatment, it's very important to review them with your oncologist to make sure none of them interferes with standard treatments.

Dee's comment:

I never tried alternative therapies. Many of these therapies offer a quick cure based on anecdotal evidence, not controlled scientific studies.

I did find that complementary therapies could help improve my quality of life by reducing the stress of dealing with a cancer diagnosis and treatment. The type of therapy that I found most useful was meditation. I would find myself getting anxious before a scan or blood test, so I found a mantra that I would repeat while taking deep breaths and it helped keep me calm.

I tried a few other complementary therapies (Nia—a combination of martial, dance and healing arts, and yoga) through classes at my local Cancer Support Community. During a Survivor's Day program at Rutgers Cancer Institute of New Jersey, I learned Jin Shin Jyutsu (a form of acupressure), which I continue to find a helpful practice.

WHAT TO DO AFTER TREATMENT IS FINISHED

45. Will the CA-125 reading ever go down to zero?

No, it usually will not go down to zero. During your treatment, we will expect that the CA-125 results will normalize, which in most laboratories is to fall below the level of 35 mg/dL. In most women, this means a fall in their CA-125 to the single digits or teens, but in others it will be slightly higher. As long as these changes stay below 35, there is usually no need to be alarmed. Remember that the CA-125 is only one part of the follow-up. It must be taken into consideration with other factors: how you are feeling, your physical examination, and if necessary, imaging tests.

In addition, at least one study shows there is no benefit to closely monitoring the CA-125 in terms of keeping the cancer from returning or increasing the chances you will live longer. This study, performed in the United Kingdom, evaluated the CA-125 in women who had completed treatment for ovarian cancer, but did not tell them what the level was. If the CA-125 rose, women were randomly assigned to immediate disclosure or to continued (and blinded) follow-up. Treatment was left to the discretion of the patient and her doctor (if the CA-125 level was disclosed) or was initiated only if there were clinical signs or symptoms of recurrence (in those in whom the levels were not revealed). With follow-up, there was no difference in survival outcomes. However, women who were notified that their CA-125 levels had increased were more likely to initiate chemotherapy earlier and experienced worse quality of life as well (probably because they started treatment earlier too).

46. How often should I be examined?

If at the end of your treatment, the cancer can't be detected, either on your physical examination, by CT scan, or by your CA-125 reading, you enter routine follow-up. Most experts agree that being seen every 3 months for the first 2 years is enough. These visits should consist of a physical assessment that includes a pelvic examination. While the value of serial testing for CA-125 is questionable, most clinicians will include CA-125 testing as a part of follow-up. In most women who have their cancer come back, the recurrence generally appears within this time frame. After 2 years, visits can be extended. If your chemotherapy isn't being administered by your surgeon, we feel it's important to continue to follow up with both your surgeon and medical oncologist at regular intervals.

47. Do I need to have CT scans as part of my regular follow-up?

There is no standard recommendation on the frequency of doing repeat CT scans. If you're doing well at your visits and there doesn't appear to be a concern that your cancer has started to grow again, there's no role for a CT scan. However, if your CA-125 reading starts to rise or goes beyond the normal range or you start to experience vague symptoms, a CT scan may be recommended.

In some women, the CA-125 is not a marker of their cancer, or it was normal at the time they were diagnosed. In such situations, more attention needs to be paid to the examination results and your symptoms, but it's reasonable to perform CT scans to reevaluate your disease at more frequent intervals, such as every 3 to 6 months.

48. When can I consider myself cured?

In women who are diagnosed with ovarian cancer and have a complete resection or an optimal debulking of their cancer, chemotherapy is done with the intent to cure. Unfortunately, there's no guarantee that you'll be cured. We do know that 80% of women will initially respond to treatment, but only around 30% will not have their cancer return. In clinical studies, we often use an arbitrary time point to determine "cure," and this is 5 years. Once you get past the 5-year mark, the likelihood of the cancer returning becomes lower and lower, and the chances of your living through the cancer become better and better.

49. Do I still need yearly mammograms?

We always recommend continued health maintenance examinations once patients complete treatment. This is because the risk of a second cancer is higher in patients who have already had one type of cancer. So, yes, you will still need a mammogram. Other health maintenance tests that you and your doctor should discuss are a screening colonoscopy and a bone density test (especially if you had both ovaries removed and are not on estrogen replacement, as there is an increased risk for osteoporosis).

50. What do I tell my family?

This is an incredibly personal question, but honesty should be the driving principle. Often, the best intentions of trying to protect your loved ones result in feelings of isolation and loneliness on the patient's part, and a sense of helplessness and distance on the part of those of us who love them. Cancer is not a diagnosis that affects only one person; it will affect everyone around you. Instead of trying to handle it alone, take advantage of the support that is likely to be available from family and friends.

51. What insurance and financial concerns must I address after my diagnosis?

It is important for you to review your health insurance policy to ensure you are covered for surgery, medical treatment, and, if necessary, second or even third consultations. Navigating the medical system can be both frustrating and time-consuming, so it is worthwhile to seek out financial help, which may be available in the financial services office of your hospital or by speaking directly to a representative of your insurance policy. You will need to know for what and where you are covered. If you find a doctor that you feel comfortable with who is not a practicing provider within your insurance plan, make sure you know what, if anything, will be covered by your primary insurance, and what portion of the bills you are likely to be personally responsible for. Your providers should be able to direct you toward the right people to speak with when it comes to billing so you can have some estimate of the charges you may incur from surgery and, if applicable, from medical treatment.

PART FOUR

Coping with Treatment-Related Side Effects

Should I take special precautions
while on chemotherapy?

What kind of diet should I follow while on
treatment? What about after treatment?

Will I be able to tolerate treatment
if I am older?

More...

52. Should I take special precautions while on chemotherapy?

Many people are under the impression that chemotherapy will require them to live in their homes unable to eat fresh fruit, enjoy flowers, other people, the movies, or even their own children or grandchildren. Yes, chemotherapy requires some diligence in terms of monitoring your own temperature if you feel warm or suspect a fever, but a woman doesn't need to change her entire life and surroundings due to the type of chemotherapy we use for ovarian cancer. The reason that many of these precautions are taken is to avoid any risk of infection when you are most vulnerable after chemotherapy, which is when your white counts decrease (called neutropenia) and you are prone to develop infections and fever. This time at risk is variable depending on what cancer you have and the regimen being used to treat it. People undergoing treatment for leukemia or who have had a bone marrow transplant are most at risk because the periods of neutropenia are very long. Fortunately, for women being treated for ovarian cancer this time is not long-lasting; in general it lasts less than a week. Therefore, they do not need to undergo this degree of protection.

Dee's comment:

How and what you tell your family and children depends on your particular situation. One of my children was a sophomore in college, and the other was a recent college graduate at the time of my initial diagnosis. Because they were older we were able to tell them exactly the reason why I was having surgery and what to expect while in treatment. Even though they were adults I still worried about telling them. And I also worried how my cancer would affect their lives.

My children were very supportive when I lost my hair, and preferred seeing me in a scarf than in a wig. My sister-in-law told her two young girls (age 7 and 9 years at the time) that I had lost my hair because I was taking medicine that would make me feel better in a few months. When we visited them they were not surprised at all that I didn't have any hair and was wearing a scarf.

You are the best judge of how, when, and how much information to share with your children, but there are organizations like Cancer Support Community and LiveSTRONG that have brochures and can provide advice on how to broach the subject with children of different ages.

53. What kind of diet should I follow while on treatment? What about after treatment?

There's a substantial amount of information about diet and its role in healing and cancer therapy. Unfortunately, none of it has been studied to any great degree, and there aren't a lot of data to help guide us in the role of diet in cancer care. A lot of patients have heard about avoiding refined sugar or white flour, because these may contribute to cancer. The bottom line is that no studies have linked diet to chemotherapy response or to a risk of recurrence. It is probably best to eat a variety of foods in moderation and to follow a heart-healthy diet. After all, the cancer does not define the patient. You are still the same person you were before cancer, at risk for heart disease, high blood pressure, and other more common medical conditions. Treat your body well by eating a balanced diet and allow yourself the time to heal.

54. Will I be able to tolerate treatment if I am older?

Treating older patients (beyond age 60) is another evolving area of study. Earlier studies suggested that age was an important factor in the prognosis for women suffering from ovarian cancer and that older women did not do as well as younger women. This theory has been subjected to more debate as we have recognized an important bias: Older patients generally are not given the same treatment options as those offered to younger patients. In fact, older women tolerate chemotherapy as well as do younger women, and the more important factor to consider is not age but the activity you're able to perform on a daily basis (your **performance status**). It is well recognized that a sicker patient who requires 24-hour home care and cannot walk without assistance will fare worse with chemotherapy than will a healthier patient, regardless of age.

Having said this, it may be wise to tailor therapy for women past the age of 70 and for those in specific situations, such as women with an underlying neuropathy from diabetes or other causes or those having a baseline hearing loss. One option may be to administer lower doses of chemotherapy more frequently (see Question 32 on page 52).

55. Should I be taking any special vitamins?

Your doctor may recommend a multivitamin a day. Anything more than that is generally not necessary. As exists for dietary advice, a lot of information has been

Performance status

A numerical description of how a person is doing in her normal day-to-day life and whether her cancer is impacting her ability to live normally.

circulated regarding vitamin supplementation to help the immune system and even about the use of homeopathic remedies, such as coral calcium and shark cartilage. Unfortunately, there aren't a lot of data to tell whether these homeopathic remedies or vitamin supplements are actually helping you. The major goal is to stay away from things that could eventually hurt you, and you need to discuss and review fully with your doctor all nontraditional medications before you start taking them. As was discussed earlier, taking antioxidants such as vitamin E and vitamin C may be a bad thing during chemotherapy.

56. What's a growth factor? When would I need it?

Growth factors are drugs that stimulate the bone marrow to recover after chemotherapy. They are available to help stimulate your red blood cells and white blood cells.

Erythropoietin is a hormone that stimulates your body to release red blood cells. Two drugs are available that essentially act like erythropoietin, epoetin alfa (aka Procrit) and darbepoetin alfa (aka Aranesp). Both are used to treat or prevent chemotherapy-induced anemia. A growth factor may be recommended by your doctor if your hemoglobin falls below a certain level. However, it is not routinely used for most women being treated for newly diagnosed ovarian cancer. If indicated, however, your doctor would need to check your iron levels to make sure you do not have an alternative reason to be anemic.

Erythropoietin

A hormone produced by the kidneys to stimulate the release of red blood cells in the bone marrow.

Both agents are given as an injection into your skin (subcutaneously). The difference between the two agents is how long they are active in your body. Epoetin alfa has to be used either three times a week or weekly (I use it weekly) because it does not stick around any longer than 7 days. Darbepoetin alfa is designed to stick around longer and therefore can be used every 2 weeks. Studies have shown they are equally effective.

Filgrastim (Neupogen) and pegfilgrastim (Neulasta) are both used to treat low white blood cell counts from chemotherapy. If your doctor thinks you're at a high risk for this complication, it may be recommended to you as a protective move. Otherwise, you may not need it and it would be used only if you had experienced a problem with your counts, such as fevers or even infections due to low blood counts (neutropenic fever), which may require you to be hospitalized. The use of these drugs can shorten the time your white blood cell counts are low. A low white blood cell count is a risk for getting an infection, which can be very serious.

These drugs also allow you to be treated on schedule, without delays or disruption, so you can complete treatment as anticipated. Filgrastim requires a daily injection into your skin, which usually begins the day after treatment and continues for 3–5 days. Pegfilgrastim stays in your system longer (about 2 weeks), so it needs to be administered only once between chemotherapy sessions.

57. How do you control nausea? What are the different medicines used?

As stated earlier, nausea is a common side effect of the chemotherapy used to treat ovarian cancer, and in some women can be a very significant side effect. Fortunately, we have strong anti-nausea medications that can specifically treat and even prevent nausea.

Ondansetron (Zofran) and granisetron (Kytril) are very potent anti-nausea drugs. They work by blocking specific pathways for nausea that are triggered by chemotherapy and work through the nervous system protein serotonin. They are available in pill form and as an injection. One dose is administered before chemotherapy treatment and then is taken by mouth at home, usually for 3 days after chemotherapy, when you're at most risk for chemotherapy-induced nausea and vomiting. A newer agent in this class, palonosetron (Aloxi), may be recommended if the others do not work. This is available only as an injection and is useful only to prevent, not to treat, nausea.

Aprepitant (Emend) also available to prevent nausea associated with chemotherapy. It also works on the nervous system, but blocks neurokinin 1 (NK1), a protein found in the brain that causes vomiting. It is taken 1 hour before chemotherapy and then again in the morning for the next 2 days. It's used in addition to other anti-nausea drugs, such as ondansetron or granisetron.

If you are going to be treated with cisplatin, then there is a risk that you may experience nausea for more than 3 days after treatment. These delayed side effects from chemotherapy are treated with steroids—most commonly dexamethasone (Decadron). These are usually taken once or twice daily and then doses are reduced over the next 4 or 5 days, called a steroid taper.

Benzodiazepines like lorazepam (Ativan) also are used to treat nausea and vomiting, in addition to being used to treat nervousness and anxiety.

Finally, prochlorperazine (Compazine) is prescribed as a general anti-vomiting drug. It is available as a pill or as a suppository, and can be used for nausea and vomiting that occurs at any point during treatment for cancer. Some women don't particularly like it due to some of its side effects, like nervousness or jitteriness.

It's very important that your doctor be aware of how you are doing before, during, and after chemotherapy treatments. Often, with adjustments in treatment or in the medications used, nausea can be very well controlled and need not be a significant problem.

Dee's comment:

As I sat with my gynecologic oncologist discussing my future chemotherapy treatments, she started to describe the side effects I would experience while taking carboplatin and Taxol. The only thing that really bothered me was when she said I might experience nausea and vomiting. I stopped her and said that vomiting was the one thing that I just couldn't deal with. She told me that I would be given a number of different drugs to prevent that from happening. I took the drugs before, during, and for a few days after getting my chemotherapy. During the nine cycles of chemotherapy I had when I was initially diagnosed, I never once vomited.

After my recurrence, I once again received carboplatin and Taxol. This time, though, the drugs I had taken previously did not prevent the nausea as well. I called the nurse help line, described how I felt, and she quickly switched me to a different drug that did the trick.

58. What can I do about the chemotherapy-related numbness and tingling?

During treatment, you will be asked about problems with numbness or tingling (**sensory neuropathy**). These can occur due to the taxanes or to cisplatin. Make sure your doctor knows if this develops and, more importantly, make sure it is being followed on treatment because it can get progressively worse. If not addressed early on, it can get so bad that it may affect your ability to do fine movements, such as buttoning your blouse, turning a door knob, or operating a can opener.

Sensory neuropathy

Numbness and tingling, usually involving the hands and feet.

If symptoms develop, there are medications that you can take to help prevent it from getting worse, and you should discuss them with your doctor. Some patients benefit from taking a vitamin called glutamine, available at most natural food stores or vitamin shops. Others get relief from the pain associated with neuropathy with the use of gabapentin (Neurontin). If your symptoms worsen, your doctor may manage them by reducing the dose of paclitaxel or switching to another drug altogether, docetaxel, which has less risk of causing neuropathy. One study done in Europe showed that docetaxel with carboplatin was as effective as paclitaxel with carboplatin, so you should not worry about such a change decreasing your chances of beating ovarian cancer.

59. Can I work while receiving treatment?

Although the treatment for ovarian cancer is very tolerable, it is generally a good idea to take some time off work when you start treatment, particularly if you choose to go through intraperitoneal (IP) treatment. IP therapy is a complicated process and may require you to be hospitalized for a portion of treatment.

For those patients on intravenous chemotherapy, some may be relatively unaffected by their treatment and will be able to work while on therapy, but others will find that they do.

60. Will I still be able to care for my kids while receiving chemotherapy? What about my pets?

You should be able to carry out most normal activities even while on chemotherapy. You should not put aside your goals and needs. In fact, most studies show that some people feel better on treatment than they did when they were diagnosed. You need not sequester yourself from your family or your pets while receiving treatment. You may be more tired, particularly as you near completion of your treatment, and may need some help in taking care of your pets or home responsibilities. However, with a little help from your friends and family, you should be able to continue your normal routines. This means, however, that you must accept help when it's offered. Many people politely refuse an offer from a friend or family member, thinking they don't want to burden others with their illness, but this habit only makes your difficult task of recovery more difficult than it needs to be. If your family and friends want to help, let them!

61. Can I still enjoy sex and intimacy, even if I have cancer treatment?

Female sexual health is a multidimensional construct that includes body image, want of intimacy, desire, arousal, orgasm, and satisfaction. It is not merely intercourse. Cancer and the treatments for ovarian cancer can disrupt many areas of female sexual health. Most prominently, a woman's vagina can thin considerably and be prone to irritation, especially if she was not in menopause at the time of surgery.

A common concern after cancer is pain with sexual intercourse, called genital pelvic pain/penetration syndrome. If not evaluated, it can lead to a domino effect on women's sexual health, and can lead to a loss of desire and reduced arousal.

However, with medical care and a patient partner, it is common to rediscover intimacy and one's sexual self. Your medical team can help in this area, but it requires an open and honest discussion about sexuality. Medication, such as vaginal estrogen in low doses, vaginal dilators, and lubrication aids, are available to help you maintain or rediscover a satisfying sexual life. In addition, some centers may have an Oncology Sexual Health specialist (or at least access to resources on this topic) to help you address this very important aspect of life. Remember, the notion that "at least you're alive" is no longer enough. Despite cancer, one deserves a fulfilling life, both sexuality and intimacy.

62. Taking my ovaries has suddenly made me have hot flashes. Is this menopause? What can I do for relief?

Removal of the ovaries will obviously result in a significant decrease of estrogen and progesterone from the circulation. A consequence of that is menopause, which sometimes may be symptomatic; patients may have hot flashes, night sweats, mood changes, and vaginal discomfort with burning and painful intercourse. The treatment of symptomatic menopause is best achieved with hormone replacement therapy. Hormone replacement therapy is usually given as a tablet, a skin patch, or a local vaginal cream or vaginal tablet, depending on the symptoms and the area that needs to be treated.

Patients who have had a total hysterectomy and who need hormone replacement therapy can be treated with estrogen alone. Hormone replacement therapy is usually safe in the setting of ovarian carcinoma; however, it should be reserved for patients who have significant menopause-related symptoms.

The lowest dose of estrogen and the shortest duration needed to help alleviate the symptoms should be used, because long-term use of hormone replacement therapy may be associated with side effects such as increased risk of breast cancer or venous thromboembolism. The decision of whether to take hormone replacement therapy will depend on a thorough discussion with your gynecologic oncologist or medical oncologist; however, if your symptoms are severe, a low-dose hormone replacement therapy may significantly improve the symptoms and improve your quality of life.

63. Is depression common after treatment?

Yes, depression is a common experience for women with ovarian cancer. Once a woman is diagnosed, she may work through a whole gamut of emotions like terror, fear, anxiety, and worry. However, as many women begin therapy, a sense of resolve and a determination to do whatever is necessary to beat the cancer soon sets in. Yet, as much as a woman looks forward to completing treatment, it is not uncommon for many to feel a sense of depression after treatment has been completed. It is often due to a sense of anxiety that nothing is being done once treatment is over (entering the "watchful waiting" period), and with that, a loss of control over what the future may hold. Many women can work through this with the passage of time, as they become more used to the frequent schedule of follow-up visits. But for some, the end of therapy brings about a sense of sadness and a sometimes overwhelming fear, which can be quite debilitating. If this appears to be occurring, it is very important to discuss such concerns with your physician. After all, no woman diagnosed with ovarian cancer should live the rest of her life paralyzed by fear or depression over what may be.

Dee's comments:

I am a "glass is half full" type of person, but while having to deal with a cancer diagnosis it is just not possible to be positive and upbeat all the time. It is a life changer.

Many people outside of my immediate family might have only seen me when I was feeling good, had energy, and was up for being out and social. My family knew and experienced a few down times with me. Hearing that I needed three more chemotherapy treatments, in addition to the six I had already just had, made me want to throw in the towel. But my faith and having my family and friends to support me through that tough time made it possible to continue.

I also found that reaching out to others diagnosed with ovarian cancer helped me. When I was initially diagnosed I called the Cancer Hope Network, and was matched with a 7-year, stage III ovarian cancer survivor who lived in my state. It meant the world to me to speak to a woman who made it past the 5-year mark and was living life to the fullest.

The hardest part of my cancer journey emotionally was when I finished treatment and saw my doctor less frequently. I felt adrift and afraid that my cancer would come back. I didn't want to share my fears and anxiety with my family because I didn't want to upset them or make them worry. That is when I found two in-person gynecologic cancer support groups: one at my cancer center and one at Cancer Support Community. To this day the women in these groups and the social worker moderator listen to my concerns, and they "get it."

If you are sad or seem to be unable to do anything for more than 2–3 weeks, be sure to tell your doctor—our emotional health is as important as our physical health.

64. When will my hair grow back?

Once you complete treatment with paclitaxel, your hair should start growing back, but certainly you should have noticeable hair growth within 3 months of stopping treatment. It may take 6 months, or even longer, to have shoulder-length hair. Do not be surprised or shocked if your hair grows back different in texture, style, or color. It may begin as gray or even white, and in more than a few women, it has come back curly. As you get farther out from treatment, your hair should resume its normal appearance as it was before you started therapy. But patience will be necessary before you get to that point.

Dee's comments:

I took everyone's advice to get my hair cut short before chemotherapy. The day before I started chemotherapy I visited a shop not far from my home to buy a wig. My doctor had given me a prescription for a "hair prosthesis" so most of the cost of the wig was covered by my insurance. I tried to get a color close to my normal color and style close to the way I wore my hair.

About 2 weeks after starting chemo my hair started falling out. What I did not expect was that my scalp would hurt. The best way to describe it is how your head feels after having your long hair in a ponytail all day. Eventually the pain did go away.

I know many women are very upset about loosing their hair but I never really felt that way. I thought if the chemo was causing my hair to fall out, then that was good because it must be doing its job on those ovarian cancer cells too.

Even though I had a wig in the months of treatment, I only wore it five times. For me the wig was too scratchy, and I was always worried that it would come off. Instead, I took to wearing fleece and wool caps during the cold winter months in New Jersey and scarves when the weather turned milder. What I did use was what is called a "halo," a hairpiece that is a ring of hair. That way when I wore my hat or scarf a little bit of hair was visible.

The other thing that I did to make myself feel better about wearing hats and scarves was to buy what I called "funky" earrings. I usually wore post earrings but I began to wear 1–2 inch long earrings with lots of colorful beads. I thought people could focus on my earrings instead of my scarf-covered head.

By about 2 month after the end of chemo my hair was long enough— more like peach fuzz—to go without a hat or scarf. When my hair did start to grow in, it grew in very curly. Curly hair was something I actually enjoyed for the relatively short period of time I had it. I always had very straight hair and spent lots of time trying to curl it. As my hair grew in, it did eventually straighten.

65. Does chemotherapy affect your memory?

A common complaint in women being treated with chemotherapy is a decrease in memory, sometimes called "chemo-brain." They complain of an inability to retain short-term memories, like what they just talked about with friends or where they put their keys. These problems can impact on their daily lives, especially if they take care of a household or are doing a mentally demanding task. Still, it is important to realize that these issues are poorly understood, and chemotherapy-induced changes in memory have not been identified in recent studies.

Dee's comments:

Sometimes my toes still tingle and my digestive system had to find a new normal, but the side effect that continues to bother me the most is "chemo brain." For me, "chemo brain" is not being able to retrieve the correct word or name for things. I will spend time describing what the object or event is because I am unable to find the right word. Sometimes a few minutes later the word will come to me. At other times, if I am lucky— my family or friends will fill in the missing word.

I deal with "chemo brain" by taking notes during important conversations, to which I can refer later to find the right words. I've also learned to build in time to rewrite my blog posts (I leave blank spaces in the post when I can't find the word). I have found that when I try to do more than one thing at a time is when I have a harder time finding the right words. So I try not to multi-task as often as I used to.

66. Will I ever enjoy my own life again?

There is no question that being diagnosed with ovarian cancer will change your life. But this does not mean it must be for the worse. Many women find a renewed sense of self after treatment ends, but it does not happen instantaneously. Instead, it is a process that might extend many months, and is often termed as the discovery of a "new normal."

Having said this, it is also common for women to suffer from anxiety over what the future may hold. However, even in this case, time is the best medicine. As you get farther and farther out from treatment, the follow-ups, the blood tests, and the radiology exams become routine, and you will be able to find a balance between the "worry" and the "rest of your life" that works best for you.

So, yes, you will be able to enjoy life, but it is essential that you give yourself time to recover from the cancer experience. Manage your own expectations and those of the people in your personal and your professional life.

PART FIVE

Symptom Management

How does ovarian cancer cause abdominal pain?

What can I do for constipation?

How do I manage pain?

More...

67. How does ovarian cancer cause abdominal pain?

Ovarian cancer may cause abdominal or pelvic pain for a variety of reasons. The pain may be related to a large ovarian mass that is pulling on the ligaments inside you or sometimes the mass can twist (torsion) and that will cause severe pain. The other causes of pain or pressure may be related to the ovarian tumor; to an abdominal tumor pressing on other organs such as the bladder, the rectum, or the intestine; or to internal bleeding related to the tumor. Obviously, if there is a large volume of tumor inside the abdomen with ascites (fluid) or bulky upper abdominal disease, this may cause pressure on the intestines or stomach and will cause pain and discomfort. The symptoms of ovarian cancer may be subtle and mild; however, any change in abdominal symptoms or bloating or indigestion should be reported to your physician promptly.

If you develop abdominal pain, it's very important that you immediately consult with your physician or seek care in an emergency room to find a reason for your pain and specifically to rule out an intestinal obstruction. The evaluation will require a physical examination and imaging studies, usually abdominal x-rays and a CT scan of your abdomen and pelvis. Intestinal obstruction, a very common complication of advanced or recurrent ovarian cancer, may require surgery.

If your physician believes that you might have an obstruction, you will have to go to the hospital. Your doctor may recommend surgery to correct the obstruction. If your pain is severe, you may require morphine or another type of narcotic, which may be offered to you as an infusion pump that allows you to control directly the amount of pain medication you get (**patient-controlled analgesia**).

It's important to realize that abdominal pain does not automatically mean that you have an obstruction. There are other possible causes for pain, and most of them can be managed without having to admit you to the hospital. Some common causes are constipation, kidney stones, or a urinary tract infection. However, an obstruction may become an emergency, and then it requires immediate evaluation to rule it out.

68. What can I do for constipation?

Constipation is a very common complaint for women with ovarian cancer. It is typically present at diagnosis and can persist throughout treatments and recurrence. Because ovarian cancer tends to grow along the surface of your bowels, the normal function of the bowels is affected, which results in constipation. You may require the use of laxatives and stool softeners, such as senna and Colace. If constipation is related to pain medications or progression of your cancer, these may not work well enough. Your doctor may recommend other medications, including lactulose, magnesium citrate, and enemas, to help with bowel movements.

69. How do I manage pain?

A primary goal of anyone involved in the treatment of cancer patients is to alleviate pain. It is always important for your doctor to perform a history of the pain, exam, and diagnostic studies to determine the source of your

Patient-controlled analgesia (PCA)

A method of providing pain medication through the vein that allows direct control over the amount required to make one comfortable.

SYMPTOM MANAGEMENT

pain. If it is related to your cancer, often it is relieved as the cancer shrinks with chemotherapy. However, the use of narcotics is often essential to help with pain. If your doctor is unsure how to dose your pain medication or if the pain is not being controlled accurately, there are now specialists in pain management whom you can see. If the pain is found to be due to a specific site of cancer that is pressing on nerves, your doctor may even recommend radiation to help relieve the pain.

70. Will the fatigue end after treatment? What can I do for it?

Fatigue is a common side effect of chemotherapy, drug therapy, and the cancer itself. Many women find their own personal way of coping with it. Perhaps one of the best treatments is to remain as active as you can. Walking daily or light exercise can often improve fatigue and other symptoms, such as insomnia. It is also good for your overall health. So, try your best to stay active, even though it may be difficult at first. You may find it becomes easier with time. Your medical team should also look for any correctable causes of fatigue, including low blood counts, dehydration, and medications (such as pain medications).

71. How do I manage the distress that comes with ovarian cancer? Does palliative care play a role?

Perhaps one of the most important messages we can provide is to find an outlet for your emotions. It is not good to keep them inside, because those feelings will find some way of coming to the surface. Yes, you must bring your own personal strength to the treatments for cancer, but you don't have to be a superhero. Accept your limitations, cry when you need to, and ask for help when you cannot do it alone. Remember that women before you have walked the same road, and as such, consider yourself part of an exclusive club that you never imagined you'd join. But you are a part of a community of women with and survivors of ovarian cancer. If help is needed, all you must do is reach out.

If you are experiencing severe symptoms of anxiety, sadness, or distress, it may be worthwhile for you to see a palliative care specialist. These clinicians are skilled in helping one cope with cancer and identifying and treating the symptoms that are causing the most bother. In addition, involving palliative care can help one live longer; at least one randomized trial of patients with advanced lung cancer showed that those who had palliative care survived longer than those who did not.

PART SIX

Relapse

How can my ovarian cancer come back if my ovaries have already been removed?

What happens if the cancer comes back?

How do you make a diagnosis of recurrence?

More...

72. How can my ovarian cancer come back if my ovaries have already been removed?

Ovarian cancer cells can escape outside the ovary and be present in many parts of the pelvic and abdominal cavity, particularly in the lining of the peritoneum. They can hide in lymph nodes in any part of your body, or even can show up as microscopic cells in your lung, liver, bone, or brain. Removal of the ovaries will ensure that the original site of cancer is removed, but it does not guarantee that the cancer will not show up elsewhere in your body.

At the time of diagnosis, you may have a small but undetectable volume of cancer cells floating throughout your peritoneum and your entire body; if not treated, these cells may grow and eventually present as a tumor recurrence. This is why most patients with ovarian cancer should receive postsurgical (or adjuvant) chemotherapy. It's a way to secure the destruction of any potential "microscopic metastasis" that may have escaped the ovaries.

73. What happens if the cancer comes back?

If ovarian cancer recurs, your treatment will depend on where the cancer is found and the length of the interval away from chemotherapy (also known as the **platinum free interval**, or **PFI**). The PFI is usually measured from the date of the last chemotherapy treatment after your initial surgery to the date of recurrence. In general, if your cancer comes back and requires treatment with another round of chemotherapy within 6 months (after you completed the prior treatment), it's considered unlikely to respond to another round of platinum-based

Platinum-free interval (PFI)

The time between the end of one chemotherapy regimen and initiation of a subsequent therapy for recurrent disease.

chemotherapy, sometimes referred to as platinum resistance. Your oncologist will generally offer you other chemotherapy drugs that work in a different way, so-called **second-line chemotherapy**. Patients whose disease returns after a short time will generally not do as well as those who have a recurrence after a year or more. If ovarian cancer recurs more than 6 months after you complete your chemotherapy, treatment will be based on where the cancer has reappeared and on your PFI. Occasionally, recurrent ovarian cancer can be cured with a combination of multimodality treatment that involves surgery, chemotherapy, and even radiation.

Second-line chemotherapy

Chemotherapy given during recurrence.

RELAPSE

74. How do you make a diagnosis of recurrence?

As mentioned earlier, women in follow-up for ovarian cancer are usually seen every 3 to 4 months and followed by physical examination and CA-125. If your cancer recurs, you will usually present with symptoms, such as abdominal swelling, increased tiredness, inability to eat, or changes in your bowel function. Sometimes they will be similar to how you originally presented. If there is a clinical suspicion of disease recurrence, a CA-125 and imaging are very important parts of the work-up. The CA-125 measure should be interpreted as a guide that you and your physician can use to monitor the activity of your cancer. The absolute number is not as important as how rapidly it's changing. Studies now show that the rate at which the CA-125 measurement doubles above normal is an important predictor of disease growth.

A rising CA-125 can be the first sign of a recurrence. Often, it precedes the cancer's showing up on a CT scan by 2 to 3 months or even longer. A recent small study from Johns Hopkins suggested that even changes within the normal range of the CA-125 measure were predictive of recurrent disease. Changes of 50% to 100% of the smallest value were a strong predictor of recurrent disease. The situation in which the CA-125 reading is elevated without any other evidence of cancer is called a **serological relapse**. If you have no symptoms of recurrence outside of the CA-125, then you and your oncologist need to determine what treatment is best for you. Currently there is no real standard of how to treat women who have a serological relapse—some women proceed with chemotherapy to get to a normal CA-125 again, whereas others undergo close observation with monthly serum CA-125s or treatment using anti-estrogen medications such as tamoxifen.

Serological relapse

Diagnosis of recurrence solely based on an elevation of a tumor marker without evidence of recurrence by radiology tests.

Dee's comments:

As with other women diagnosed with the disease, my doctor developed a follow-up plan for me. It helped to know that I would be followed with scans, physical exams, and blood work. The further out I was from my diagnosis, the less frequent are the doctor visits.

Two and a half years after finishing my initial chemotherapy, two tumors appeared on my CT scan, one on my liver and one on my spleen. Because my progression-free interval was greater than 6 months, I was considered platinum sensitive. I was offered a number of options: surgery then chemotherapy (carboplatin and Taxol, C&T), chemotherapy (C&T) then surgery, or a clinical trial, which would randomize me to surgery first and then chemotherapy (C&T) and Avastin, or vice versa.

I felt strongly about having the surgery first if it was offered, so that is the option I chose. During the surgery they examined all areas of the abdomen and pelvis and no other visible cancer was found. I followed the surgery 2 months later with C&T until I had a severe allergic reaction to the carboplatin. I finished the last four treatments with Taxol only.

75. When is surgery indicated after a relapse?

This is a very important question because new and emerging data suggest that a large percentage of patients with recurrent ovarian carcinoma may benefit from reoperation and removal of this tumor prior to more treatment with chemotherapy or even radiation therapy. The choice of women for a "secondary cytoreduction" or repeat surgery to remove recurrent cancer depends on the following selection criteria:

- Your disease-free interval; in other words, how many months since stopping the first treatment you have been without evidence of disease before this recurrence was identified
- Whether the recurrence involves a single site or multiple sites in the body
- Whether there is disease throughout your abdomen or pelvis (also called carcinomatosis)

In general, patients must be medically fit to undergo surgery and without an obvious contraindication to a laparotomy, which is an open procedure in the abdomen or pelvis. At Memorial Sloan-Kettering Cancer Center, the general selection criteria to offer secondary cytoreduction for recurrent ovarian carcinoma include patients with a single site of recurrence that has occurred at least 6 months since the completion of chemotherapy—in other words, a disease-free interval of at least 6 months. In fact, the longer the disease-free interval, the better the outcome is for these patients. This single site of recurrence may be in the pelvis or the abdomen or sometimes the liver or the lung. Usually, patients who have a single site of recurrent ovarian carcinoma may benefit from secondary cytoreductive surgery where this tumor is removed, particularly if the disease-free interval is long.

Patients who have multiple sites of recurrences but no obvious carcinomatosis may also benefit from secondary cytoreduction, particularly if the disease-free interval is greater than one year. Patients who have carcinomatosis and large ascites are the least likely to benefit from secondary cytoreduction; however, there may be a role in highly selected patients: those women with carcinomatosis but with a disease-free interval of more than 30 months after their completion of primary chemotherapy.

In summary, patients who have recurrent ovarian carcinoma may benefit significantly from discussing whether a secondary surgery may be of benefit in their disease. This discussion is best held with a gynecologic oncologist. As our understanding of the management of recurrent ovarian carcinoma improves, more and more patients may benefit from repeat surgery for recurrent disease, particularly if the disease-free interval is greater than one year and the recurrence is isolated to a single site or to a few sites without evidence of carcinomatosis.

76. If the cancer comes back, can I still be cured?

Most women who experience a recurrence can no longer realistically expect to be cured. Rarely, a patient may be found to have recurrence in only one area within the pelvis. In this kind of situation, using a combination of surgery, chemotherapy, and radiation, oncologists can once again treat the disease with the hope of a long remission.

In those patients whose tumor recurs and is found in multiple areas of their abdomen or pelvis (or both) or whose disease has traveled to their lungs, liver, or elsewhere, the cancer is not curable. There is effective treatment that may be able to reduce the volume of disease and even put your disease back into remission. However, a remission does not last for long, and you will likely be in and out of treatment for the rest of your life.

If you're dealing with recurrent cancer, you must refocus your mind from "getting a cure" for the disease to ways of "living with it." Physicians may make the analogy that ovarian cancer is like diabetes. Although both can be fatal if not treated appropriately, neither should be considered a death sentence, and the potential for living productive lives despite these diagnoses really does exist.

Fortunately, a number of drugs are available to treat ovarian cancer. In fact, physicians can even use some drugs (the taxanes, particularly) at different doses and schedules successfully. With appropriate use of these drugs, allowing for **treatment holidays** when the cancer appears to be under control, patients can expect to live for years.

RELAPSE

Treatment holiday

A break in treatment that allows the body time to recover from toxicity.

77. What treatments are available if my cancer comes back? What does it mean to have platinum-sensitive or platinum-resistant recurrent cancer?

If your cancer comes back despite first-line (or adjuvant) treatment, there are multiple options still available. The choice will depend largely on your platinum-free interval (PFI).

PFI 6 months or longer. Patients who had a PFI of at least six months are referred to as having **platinum-sensitive** recurrent ovarian cancer and re-treatment with a combination platinum-based regimen is often recommended. A vast majority of these patients will respond once more to platinum, and many can be placed back in to remission. In addition, the option of surgery should always be considered (see Question 75 on page 105).

Carboplatin can be used in combination with other chemotherapies, including paclitaxel, pegylated liposomal doxorubicin, and gemcitabine. A choice between them is often based on patient, provider, and practical considerations. For example, if someone had a difficult time with numbness after paclitaxel, then re-treatment with paclitaxel might not be the best choice. Instead, carboplatin plus pegylated liposomal doxorubicin might be used instead.

In addition to chemotherapy, combination treatment may also include the angiogenesis inhibitor, bevacizumab. One trial compared carboplatin plus gemcitabine with or without bevacizumab and showed that use of bevacizumab delayed disease progression more effectively. However, there was no difference in overall

Platinum-sensitive

Term used to describe women with recurrent ovarian cancer who recurred six months or longer after the end of prior treatment with a platinum agent (e.g., carboplatin).

survival whether or not the 3-drug or 2-drug combination was used.

Unlike the first-line setting, it is hard to predict how much treatment you will need. Your doctor may recommend *at least* six cycles, but more often than not, the duration of treatment will depend on how you are tolerating treatment and how well it is keeping your cancer under control. While six cycles might be sufficient, for some women, more cycles will be recommended.

For patients who achieve their best response to platinum-based therapy, your doctor might discuss continuation of treatment (sometimes called maintenance therapy). Unfortunately, there are no good data to show that maintenance chemotherapy improves outcomes for women with platinum-sensitive ovarian cancer. However, for a select group of patients with ovarian cancer associated with a BRCA mutation, a large trial showed that using the PARP inhibitor, olaparib, can significantly prolong the interval before cancer starts progressing (called **progression-free survival**). In Europe, olaparib has been recommended for approval for this indication by their regulatory agency. This indication has not been approved in the United States; instead, olaparib is approved for use in women with a BRCA mutation who have progressed after multiple lines of treatment.

PFI < 6 months. Women who experience remission for less than six months are referred to as having **platinum-resistant** recurrent disease. For these patients, treatment that can control disease and cause the least amount of toxicities are the tenets of care. In addition, platinum is rarely re-administered because the chance of a response is not that high.

RELAPSE

Progression-free survival

The time interval between the start of a treatment and when the disease starts to grow once more.

Platinum-resistant

Term used to describe women with recurrent ovarian cancer who relapse less than six months after the end of prior platinum-based treatment.

It is important that the goals of treatment be clear for you. Cure is not realistic, so it often requires a shift from "beating cancer" to "living with cancer." Treatment should be aimed at keeping the cancer from *progressing* because limited data suggest that women do just as well if their cancer stopped growing (or was stable) or if it responded to treatment. One can live with cancer, and live well. Treatment should never be worse than the disease itself.

Fortunately, many drugs that are active in treating ovarian cancer can be tried. These include liposomal doxorubicin (Doxil), topotecan (Hycamtin), gemcitabine (Gemzar), docetaxel (Taxotere), vinorelbine (Navelbine); hexamethylamine (Hexalen); and etoposide (VePesid; see **Table 5**). As mentioned above, the choice of treatment can be tailored based on any prior treatment-related toxicities you experienced (or may still be experiencing), your preferences, and your goals.

In addition to chemotherapy, bevacizumab is an active drug for the treatment of platinum-resistant ovarian cancer. In one trial, single-agent chemotherapy (pegylated liposomal doxorubicin, paclitaxel, gemcitabine, or topotecan) was administered with or without bevacizumab. Treatment with chemotherapy plus bevacizumab was significantly better and resulted in higher response rates and longer durations of progression-free survival. In addition, it appeared that bevacizumab might also improve overall survival. Based on these results, the U.S. Food and Drug Administration (FDA) approved bevacizumab for use in women with platinum-resistant ovarian cancer, when coupled with chemotherapy.

Table 5 Standard Agents for Ovarian Cancer

Agent	Activity	Route of Infusion	Major Side Effects
Platinum analogs	Cross-link DNA, lead ultimately to DNA damage and cell death		
Cisplatin[1]		By vein every 3 weeks	Nausea, vomiting; numbness, tingling that may not be reversible; kidney injury; hearing loss; ringing in the ears (tinnitus)
Carboplatin[1]		By vein every 3 weeks	Lowered platelet count and white blood cell count; possible infection; nausea (less than with cisplatin); mild numbness, tingling; low risk for hearing problems
Taxanes	Inhibits cells from dividing by binding microtubules		
Paclitaxel[1]		By vein either as 1-hour infusion weekly; 3-hour infusion (if given with carboplatin) every 3 weeks; or 24-hour infusion every 3 weeks (if given with cisplatin)	Allergic reactions; complete hair loss; muscle and joint pain; numbness, tingling (reversed when drug is stopped); lowers white cell count
Docetaxel[2]		By vein as 1-hour infusion, every week or every three weeks.	Allergic reactions; lowered white cell count; hair loss; diarrhea; fluid retention

(continues)

Table 5 Standard Agents for Ovarian Cancer (continued)

Agent	Activity	Route of Infusion	Major Side Effects
Vinca alkaloids	Stop cells from multiplying by binding cell structures called tubulin		
Vinorelbine[2]		By vein every 2–3 weeks (vincristine, vinblastine); every 1–2 weeks (vinorelbine)	Skin and soft-tissue damage from leaks into skin; numbness, tingling; constipation (severe with vinblastine); nausea; hair loss; lowered white blood cells
Topoisomerase inhibitors	Stabilize DNA with enzyme (topoisomerase), leads to DNA damage and cell death		
Topotecan[1]		By vein weekly or daily for 5 days every 3 weeks	Lowered red and white blood cells, platelets; hair loss, fatigue, or rash (less common)
Etoposide[2]		Orally for 3 of 4 weeks	Lowered white blood cells and platelets; nausea, vomiting; hair loss; leukemia reported in women previously treated with etoposide
Anthracycline antibiotics	Interrupts DNA, leads to cell death		
Doxorubicin[1]		By vein every 3 weeks	Serious tissue injury from intravenous line leak; lowered white blood cells, platelets; heart failure
Pegylated Liposomal doxorubicin[1]		By vein every 4 weeks	Painful rash on palms and soles; acute infusion reaction (flushing, chills, back pain, shortness of breath, lowered blood pressure), generally resolves with interruption of infusion

RELAPSE

Agent	Activity	Route of Infusion	Major Side Effects
Antimetabolites	Incorporates into DNA and leads to DNA damage and cell death		
Gemcitabine[2]		By vein weekly for 3 of 4 weeks	Lowered white blood cells, platelets; rash; shortness of breath; flu-like syndrome; mild nausea
Antitumor antibiotics			
Bleomycin[2]	Breaks DNA in presence of copper, iron, and cobalt; causes cell death	By vein weekly	Lung toxicity (possibly fatal); fever; oral ulcers; hair loss; skin darkening; anorexia; lowered blood cell counts
Alkylating agents	Disrupt DNA, cause cell death		
Cyclophosphamide[1]		By vein every 3 weeks	Nausea, vomiting; lowered blood cell counts; bladder bleeding (hemorrhagic cystitis); hair loss
Angiogenesis inhibitors	Inhibits new blood vessel formation by blocking the vascular endothelial growth factor (VEGF) receptor		
Bevacizumab[1]		By vein every 2 or every 3 weeks	Hypertension; proteinuria; bleeding; poor wound healing; risk of bowel perforation
Poly-ADP ribose polymerase (PARP) inhibitors	Inhibits enzyme important for the repair of DNA. Specifically indicated for patients with a known BRCA mutation.		
Olaparib[1]		By mouth, twice daily	Nausea, vomiting, fatigue, dyspepsia or dysgeusia

[1] FDA approved for use in ovarian cancer.

[2] Approved for other uses but sometimes prescribed off-label for ovarian cancer.

It is important at this point to clarify how drugs are prescribed. There are three types of drugs that might be used to treat ovarian cancer. The first kind is the experimental drugs, which have not been approved for use by the FDA and cannot be prescribed outside of a clinical trial, unless a physician gets a "compassionate use" waiver for a patient who has run out of options. The second kind includes all drugs that have completed clinical trials in ovarian cancer patients and were found to be effective; these drugs have been given the FDA's stamp of approval for use in ovarian cancer patients, although the approval is sometimes qualified—that is, they may be approved for use in one stage of the disease but possibly not for another. The third kind is a gray area: drugs that have been approved for use in a similar disease (for example, breast cancer) but not for ovarian cancer. Such drugs may be prescribed "off-label"—that is, not in accordance with the rather stringent FDA indications—if the physician has reason to believe they might be effective. This is not as much of a stretch as it might sound. In many cases, very similar drugs are approved for use in ovarian cancer, but the particular drug being prescribed off-label simply hasn't gotten through sufficient trials to ascertain the proper dose, its effectiveness for a given stage of cancer, or that it is more effective and/or less toxic than the standard approved drugs. Looking at Table 5, you'll see, for example, that the drug paclitaxel is approved for ovarian cancer, although docetaxel is not. Both are taxanes, and both are effective against similar cancers, so it's entirely possible that docetaxel could work against ovarian cancer—but it's not approved. Only by going through (and passing) the rigorous testing required by the FDA will it gain that approval.

78. *Is there any way to choose which chemotherapy option will work best for me?*

There are several tests currently available or in development to predict either chemotherapy resistance (which drugs are unlikely to work for you) or chemotherapy sensitivity (which drugs are more likely to be effective for you). In general, they require fresh samples (usually tumor biopsies or fluid samples from ascites or pleural effusions), which are then exposed to different drugs (and combinations of drugs) in a laboratory setting in order to see with which drugs your cancer grows despite being exposed to them (testing for resistance) or which drugs can kill it best (sensitivity). If you are predicted to be resistant to certain drugs, then your physician may avoid them because they are not likely to work.

Despite the promise of these tumor resistance assays, their role in the management of ovarian cancer remains unclear. A recent statement by the American Society of Clinical Oncology reviewed the evidence for the use of these assays and concluded that there was insufficient evidence that they improved survival. Therefore, at this point, they are considered investigational and not recommended for routine management decisions.

For women with ovarian cancer that may be associated with a genetic predisposition, especially if there is a chance a BRCA mutation might be present, testing for a BRCA mutation should be performed, so that we can determine if olaparib is a good treatment for you. In the United States, a patient must test positive on a diagnostic test that was approved at the same time that olaparib was. This test, the BRACAnalysis CX test, will determine if you are BRCA-mutation positive. If you are, then you are a candidate for olaparib. Again, in the United States, it can be used to treat women with advanced ovarian cancer, particularly if the cancer continued to progress despite three prior lines of treatment.

79. How do you decide between using a combination of drugs or single-agent chemotherapy?

Earlier, we discussed the importance of the platinum-free interval (PFI) in helping decide about re-treatment with a platinum agent (see Question 77 on page 108). For women who have platinum-resistant disease (PFI < 6 months), the standard of care is to use single agents, while for women who are platinum-sensitive (PFI 6 months or longer), platinum-based combinations are most often used.

Beyond the PFI, your clinicians should take into account how you did with prior treatment, which can help them decide which of the many options is the right one for you. In addition, whether or not you are symptomatic of the disease, or if there is a large volume of tumor present, may factor in to decisions. If you are symptomatic, you may be best treated using combination chemotherapy plus bevacizumab. This regimen appears to increase the response rates, which may hopefully help your symptoms. However, if you did not do well with prior treatment, have a lot of lingering toxicities, or are too ill for combination therapy, your clinician might decide single-agent therapy will be best, even if you have platinum-sensitive disease.

80. What are the risks with re-treatment using carboplatin?

It is recognized that between 5% and 34% of women undergoing re-treatment with carboplatin the second time around will experience an allergic reaction to carboplatin. Curiously, it often occurs during the second re-treatment cycle (or eighth cumulative cycle). The symptoms of an allergic reaction can range from mild (redness or itching) to severe (changes in blood pressure and difficulty breathing) to full-blown anaphylaxis. There is no way to predict who is going to have an allergic reaction to carboplatin, so monitoring during re-treatment is critical. If you do experience an allergic reaction to carboplatin, it does not necessarily mean you can never receive it again. However, the risks and the potential benefits of further platinum treatment should be re-evaluated to see if further treatment makes sense.

There are case reports of death during treatment with a platinum after an allergic reaction developed. Because of this, recent studies have evaluated the use of desensitization protocols with carboplatin. Desensitization describes the process of a slow and gradual re-exposure to the drug with the intent of not triggering an allergic reaction. It has been used historically as a way to re-treat penicillin-allergic patients. The same approach has been used successfully with carboplatin, and this approach is recommended if the decision is made to continue platinum therapy. However, if your reaction is very serious (anaphylaxis, for example), then carboplatin rechallenge may not be recommended.

RELAPSE

81. If my cancer goes into remission, what can I do to increase my chances that it won't come back again?

Recent data suggest that a second remission only rarely will be as long as the first. With the approval of molecularly targeted treatments, your doctor might suggest that bevacizumab be continued for up to a year (though without the chemotherapy), and if you have a BRCA mutation, your doctor might talk to you about using olaparib after chemotherapy has completed.

There are little data showing the role of maintenance chemotherapy, however. If you are interested in doing something active, you should talk to your clinicians about potential clinical trials, which are looking at different ways to prevent a recurrence, such as immunotherapy or vaccines.

82. How long will I live now that my cancer has recurred?

This question is the one nearly every patient with cancer asks (or worries about, even if she doesn't ask it), but it's almost impossible to predict how much time a specific patient will have. The fact is that some women will die quickly from their cancer, whereas others will live well beyond 5 years, and there's no predicting who will live longer and who won't. Some patients given prognoses of a few months live for years longer than their doctors expected. Most clinical trials show that survival from a diagnosis of recurrence ranges from 40% to 84% at 3 years. However, we must emphasize that many factors must be taken into consideration for each individual patient. You shouldn't try to apply these statistics to your specific cancer and situation. Remember, too, that your doctor's prognosis of "2 to 3 years" is made without any knowledge of future scientific breakthroughs. There are plenty of people alive today whose doctors predicted short lifespans for them initially—people whose lives were saved by the creation of new forms of cancer therapy that work well on even advanced cancers. So take any predictions about your future with a big grain of salt, because medicine, like everything else, changes very rapidly.

Dealing with recurrent cancer is about more than simply living as long as possible, however. An important aspect of the prognosis is knowing how much good time you have left to you, also referred to as "quality of life." We can improve and lengthen your "good-quality life" by offering chemotherapy to control your cancer from spreading and to limit cancer-related symptoms; by making sure that any pain you have is addressed fully; by using every means necessary to ensure that your bowels continue to function; and by knowing when further therapy is likely to hurt you more than help you. All this must be done in the setting of an open and honest relationship with your physician.

Dee's comments:

Hearing you have a recurrence is scary because if you are like me, you thought you would be the one to beat the odds and not suffer a recurrence. I recurred on my liver and spleen 2½ years after finishing my initial chemotherapy. After learning of this recurrence, I had some very frank conversations with my gynecologic oncologist. I learned that a "cure" may not be possible, and that I would be treating my cancer as a chronic illness. I was also told that my remission after this recurrence would most likely be shorter than my first remission.

RELAPSE

But as I have learned with this disease, every woman is different. For me, my second remission has been longer than my first. It is over 5 years now since my recurrence and I remain NED (no evidence of disease). So far there is no way to predict which women will recur and which ones will have long remissions.

PART SEVEN

If Treatment Fails

How do I know when it's time to stop treatment?

What is a PEG tube? Do I need one?

Does intravenous feeding play a role?

More...

83. How do I know when it's time to stop treatment?

The relationship between you and your oncologist is very important and must be built on honesty and trust. This becomes more and more important if you're dealing with recurrent ovarian cancer, particularly as different treatments become necessary to try to control your cancer. Because this is a cancer that can be controlled in many women, most patients will undergo several regimens of chemotherapy with the hope of sending the cancer into remission or at least stopping it from actively growing. In fact, it's not uncommon for patients to receive three or even more different types of chemotherapy during the course of their cancer.

One of the hardest questions to ask—and even harder to answer—is when to stop trying. Sometimes, a patient will become too sick for further treatment, in which case the oncologist would recommend stopping. Other times, it's the patient who refuses further treatment and instead chooses to live out the rest of her life naturally.

For the majority of patients, the time to stop may be on realizing that, after multiple rounds with different types of chemotherapy, the cancer has only continued to grow and no promising agents are being used in a clinical trial (a test involving patients and drugs). However, ultimately you and your physician must make the decision to stop. If patients in this type of situation still maintain an independent lifestyle, continuing other types of novel treatment or chemotherapy may be reasonable.

If a patient's bowels stop working, particularly if this happens after or during one of these drug regimens (programs or schedules), doctors should discontinue treatment. The reason is that chemotherapy cannot reverse a bowel obstruction. In fact, it can make things worse and cause more complications rather than helping or even making patients feel better.

84. What is a PEG tube? Do I need one?

A **PEG** tube is a **percutaneous endoscopic gastrostomy tube**. The name describes how and where it's placed. A stomach specialist or **gastroenterologist** would place it during a short procedure. Usually, your doctor would give you medication to make the insertion more comfortable, but it does not require that you be put to sleep, as with regular surgery.

During the procedure, the gastroenterologist will use a special fiber-optic camera, called an **endoscopic camera**, introduced through your mouth and into your stomach. Once it's in place, the specialist would pump air into your stomach so that when a light shines in the internal stomach, it can be seen outside, through the skin overlying it. The specialist would make a hole through the skin and into your stomach and, through this hole, would place a tube by passing it over the camera. It remains in place in your stomach and exits through the hole in your skin.

The main purpose of a PEG tube is to provide continuous stomach drainage in patients who have a **bowel obstruction** due to cancer growing around the small intestines and in whom surgery cannot be performed for technical reasons. A PEG tube is not placed in everyone who has ovarian cancer. It's usually reserved for patients whose cancer is very advanced and who suffer from continual vomiting caused by gastric juices backing up from

IF TREATMENT FAILS

Percutaneous endoscopic gastrostomy (PEG)

A tube placed by a gastroenterologist that is inserted through your skin (percutaneous) and into your stomach.

Gastroenterologist

A medical specialist in treating disorders of the esophagus, stomach, bowel, and rectum.

Endoscopic camera

A flexible camera within a tube (the endoscope) that is used to do minimally invasive procedures.

Bowel obstruction

Condition where the small or large bowel is blocked due to either adhesions or tumor that causes the bowel to back up instead of work normally (to get rid of stool).

the bowels because of an intestinal obstruction (blockage). The PEG tube allows the fluid to exit the body more easily, which helps the patient to stop vomiting.

The PEG tube is usually permanent and is attached to a drainage bag into which the stomach contents are drained continuously. Women who have PEG tubes can continue to drink liquids, but whatever is not absorbed into their bowel exits through the PEG tube, instead of coming back up as vomit. Women with PEG tubes can also enjoy independence, because the bag to which the PEG tube is attached can be attached to the patient's leg.

The PEG tube is not a treatment for cancer; it's a way to relieve vomiting due to malignant intestinal obstruction, so that you're not throwing up all the time. Sometimes, if you're feeling better, your doctor might disconnect the tube so that you can take pills and eat and drink. However, if you were suddenly to feel nauseous, the tube can be allowed to drain so that you're not throwing up.

It's important to realize that not all patients require a PEG tube. It's offered only as a way to live with the cancer when it's far advanced and the treatments are no longer keeping it under control. As a consequence, it's used only in the most advanced cases when the disease is considered terminal.

85. Does intravenous feeding play a role?

Total parenteral nutrition (TPN)

Nutrition that is given by vein.

Intravenous feeding, or **total parenteral nutrition (TPN),** is usually reserved for women when they first get sick with their cancer. Surgeons use TPN to help to provide nourishment to their patient to make the aggressive up-front treatments of surgery and chemotherapy more manageable.

However, the role of TPN for women with recurrent ovarian cancer is more controversial. If the cancer is growing to the point at which the patient can no longer eat or drink, TPN is probably of very little value. A recent study from Women & Infants' Hospital in Providence suggested that women with advanced ovarian cancer who were on TPN had a shorter overall survival time than women not receiving TPN.

Its use requires an indwelling (permanently placed) intravenous line or MediPort and can cause complications (e.g., clotting) due to the catheter, metabolic problems, and infections. More importantly, it has not been found to improve the life span of advanced cancer patients, nor has it been shown to offer much in the way of relieving hunger or thirst. In one study of patients with different types of cancer receiving TPN, patients with ovarian cancer given home TPN had the shortest survival rate, compared to similar patients with colon cancer or appendiceal primaries.

In individual situations, TPN may be offered, but that option must take place only after a thoughtful discussion among you, your family, and your doctor. Such a frank discussion should take into account the pros and cons of TPN in the context of how you're doing at the time.

86. What is hospice?

Hospice is a part of **palliative** care and signifies end-of-life care. When treatments are no longer working and the disease has become terminal, the doctor may recommend hospice. It represents a concerted effort by doctors and other health care providers to recognize that the end of life is a part of the disease process. We have a responsibility to help the patient and her family

Palliation

To provide relief of pain. Adj.: palliative.

to remain as comfortable as possible with dignity and free of pain. Hospice care can be delivered either in an inpatient facility (either a hospital or nursing home–type setting) or at home.

Often, providers make an attempt to honor the wishes of a patient. If a woman chooses to go home to live out the rest of her life, providers can set up hospice services to meet her needs and address issues of pain and comfort. They also try to take into account the concerns of her family. However, if the patient's needs are too much for the family to handle or if she's too sick to go home, her health care providers may recommend inpatient hospice. The ultimate goal is to provide a peaceful death when a patient reaches the end stages of cancer.

87. What is a DNR order?

DNR stands for "do not resuscitate." Other terms for this include Do Not Intubate (DNI) and Do Not Attempt Resuscitation (DNAR). This is a physician's order and is meant to represent your wishes in case something happens to you that, without the use of machines, you would likely die. If you were unable to speak for yourself, this order will help your family, your physician, or your health care proxy to make decisions for you when that time comes. In this order, you would be asked to state specifically what you would want done and what you would not want done if you were to have a life-threatening event.

These decisions are in large part state-determined. For example, in Connecticut, a DNR order must specify clearly if you do or do not want to have a tube inserted into your throat to help you breathe (**intubation**), cardiac resuscitation, intravenous fluids, or total parenteral

Intubation

Process by which a person is placed on a breathing machine.

nutrition (TPN). In New York, both intubation and cardiac resuscitation are included in the DNR order.

You should not wait to establish a DNR order until you become so sick that you have to make the decision without having time to really think about it or you are considered terminal. The best time to discuss it is when you are still healthy, so that you and your family can ask questions and thoroughly talk it over with your doctor.

It's important to realize that a DNR order is not permanent. If at any point you change your mind regarding what you would want for yourself in a life-threatening situation, your health care team and your family must respect your wishes.

If you opt to have a DNR in place, you should ask your doctor for an order that you can keep with you at home. In some states, this consists of a Medical Order for Life Sustaining Treatment (MOLST) or a Physician Order for Life Sustaining Treatment (POLST).

88. What is a health care proxy?

A health care proxy is a person whom you designate to make health care decisions for you in the event that you are unable to tell your physicians your wishes. This can be a very important role, so it's important for you as a patient to initiate a discussion of what you would want for yourself. Only then can your physicians make sure that they're abiding by your wishes. If you don't designate a health care proxy, your family often has to make decisions for you. Doing that can be risky because, although they may be acting with your best interests at heart, their decisions may not necessarily be what you would want. In addition, it's not uncommon for different members of your family to disagree with each other, particularly when it comes to someone they love. By designating a health care proxy, your family and loved ones would know that you specifically chose someone to speak for you.

Dee's comments:

Before my first surgery I chose my husband as my health care proxy. He knows exactly how I want to be treated when I am no longer able to communicate my wishes.

I admit it is not an easy discussion to have with family members. For me it was difficult to think of a time I would be unable to make decisions for myself. For family members it is difficult to think about a time when a loved one is so ill or nearing death. But it is a very important discussion to have. It may happen that your first choice as proxy is not available or willing to be proxy. In that case ask another family member, partner, or friend if he or she is willing to take on that role for you.

89. What are the end stages of ovarian cancer like?

Ovarian cancer usually causes problems by spreading throughout the abdomen and pelvis. Although cancer can involve the brain, lungs, and liver, most women die of disease affecting their bowels. Obstruction of the large bowel (the colon) can lead to problems with bowel movements, causing constipation. This can cause the colon to become very large, much like a balloon, also called **colonic dilation**. If it persists, it can become an emergency and result in a tear in the bowel, called a perforation. In that event, a surgeon may recommend emergency surgery to deal with the obstruction.

Colonic dilation

Swelling of the bowel due to gas or liquid that cannot move through.

The cancer can also obstruct the small bowel and result in problems when the patient tries to eat. This results in nausea and vomiting of food; if not eating, a patient may also vomit up bile. This, too, can be very painful and may require a **nasogastric (NG) tube** initially and a PEG tube (discussed in detail in Question 84) if it does not resolve.

Tumor growth in the belly can also block the flow of urine. When the urine backs up into the kidneys, the kidneys and the tubes that attach the kidneys to the bladder (the **ureters**) can become enlarged, called hydronephrosis if only the kidneys are enlarged or **hydroureteronephrosis** if the ureter is also involved. Although this condition can cause some pain, it may not cause any symptoms at all. However, it can cause the kidneys to stop working if it goes on for a long time. Other problems can include the development of channels between the bowel and the skin or bladder, called **fistulas**.

Nasogastric (NG) tube

A tube placed temporarily through the nose (naso) into the stomach (gastric) to help relieve continuous vomiting caused by a bowel obstruction.

Ureter

The anatomical structure that enables us to get rid of urine. It connects the kidney to the bladder.

Hydronephrosis

Abnormal enlargement of the kidney.

Hydroureteronephrosis

Abnormal enlargement of the kidney and the tube where urine flows, called the ureter.

Fistulas

Abnormally formed channels between two otherwise separate organs, such as between the vagina and bladder (vesicovaginal) or between the bowel and the skin (enterocutaneous).

IF TREATMENT FAILS

PART EIGHT

Prevention, Screening, and Advocacy

Can I protect myself from getting ovarian cancer?

Can I get ovarian cancer if I've had my ovaries removed?

Will fertility drugs increase my risk of ovarian cancer?

More...

PREVENTION

90. Can I protect myself from getting ovarian cancer?

The only way to prevent developing ovarian cancer is to have your ovaries removed. However, for women who want to have children or at least want the ability to have children in the future, that's not an option. Also, because this is a relatively uncommon disease, there's a strong possibility that a lot of women who would never have gotten ovarian cancer would go through the procedure unnecessarily. Right now, having your ovaries removed to prevent ovarian cancer (termed a **prophylactic oophorectomy**) is reserved for women considered to be at high risk for developing ovarian cancer. For women who are undergoing a hysterectomy for whatever reason, removing the fallopian tubes (termed a **salpingectomy**) may also effectively reduce one's risk for ovarian cancer. Although still an area being actively investigated, it is based around the theory that most ovarian cancers originate in the fallopian tube, which is discussed in Question 8 on page 14. Oral contraceptives, or birth control pills, also can provide protection against the development of ovarian cancer.

Prophylactic oophorectomy

Removal of a woman's ovaries in an attempt to reduce or remove a risk for ovarian cancer in the future.

Salpingectomy

Removal of the fallopian tube.

91. Can I get ovarian cancer if I've had my ovaries removed?

Technically speaking, having your ovaries removed will prevent you from getting ovarian cancer. However, removing your ovaries cannot **prevent primary peritoneal cancer**, which behaves similarly and is treated in the same way. It turns out that the cells that line the peritoneum are the same cells that line the ovaries. Thus, cancer can arise out of the peritoneal lining.

Primary peritoneal cancer

Cancer that arises from the lining of the gut, or the peritoneum. This cancer behaves similarly to ovarian cancer and is treated much in the same way.

Although this cancer is much rarer than ovarian cancer, having your ovaries removed can't prevent it.

92. Will fertility drugs increase my risk of getting ovarian cancer?

Although taking fertility medications is suspected of increasing one's risk of ovarian cancer by causing your ovaries to make more eggs, no conclusive evidence suggests that this is true. Certainly, there is a concern that hyperstimulation of the ovary can predispose to the development of ovarian cancer, owing to the frequent shedding of the ovarian surface, but this has yet to be proven.

SCREENING

93. Can ovarian cancer be inherited?

Yes, ovarian cancer can be inherited, but it's important to know that the majority of cases of ovarian cancer are not inherited. In fact, estimates figure that only 15–20% of all ovarian cancers are hereditary.

Generally, a hereditary cancer syndrome is suspected if, at the age of diagnosis, a patient is younger than age 40; has a history of prior breast cancer; or has a strong family history of other cancers, particularly in the immediate family. This having been said, certain well-recognized cancer syndromes run in families and are associated with an increased risk of ovarian cancer.

The most common hereditary cancer syndrome is the hereditary breast-ovarian cancer (HBOC) syndrome. If three or more cases of cancer are found within your immediate family (**first-degree relatives**) along with a

First-degree relatives

Blood relatives of your immediate family (father, mother, sister, or brother).

PREVENTION, SCREENING, AND ADVOCACY

133

history of four or more early-age breast cancer cases or a history of ovarian cancer at any age, clinically your family has an HBOC syndrome. Most of the cases of this syndrome are due to mutations in one of two genes, called *BRCA1* and *BRCA2*. The *BRCA1* gene has been found on chromosome 17; *BRCA2* is located on chromosome 13. The mutations within these genes may confer a risk for different types of cancers, but both are specifically associated with an increase in breast and ovarian cancer.

In addition to breast and ovarian cancer, these mutations are associated with an increased risk of other cancers. *BRCA1* mutation carriers may have an increased risk of colon cancer and prostate cancer (in men). *BRCA2* mutation carriers have an increased risk of male breast cancer, prostate cancer, malignant melanoma, and cancers of the pancreas, colon, gallbladder, and stomach.

Another syndrome found to exist in certain families is termed the Lynch II syndrome, which is a subtype of hereditary nonpolyposis colon cancer (HNPCC) syndrome. Such families contain multiple family members with colon cancer and cancers of the uterus. However, in addition to harboring these two, they are known to have members who have had breast cancer, ovarian cancer, and other types of cancer. These include cancers of the brain, stomach, and small bowel; leukemias; and sarcomas. The HNPCC syndrome is associated with mutations in human mismatch repair genes that are responsible for correcting errors or mutations in our DNA.

The final type of cancer syndrome associated with ovarian cancer is termed a site-specific ovarian cancer syndrome. This syndrome is seen in families with multiple members who develop only ovarian cancer. Researchers have not completely worked out the genetic explanation for this syndrome, although a proportion of these tumors may end up being due to BRCA-related mutations. Although these families' members have only ovarian cancer, their female members are still considered at risk for breast cancer. Recent data suggest that the opposite may not be true—women with a strong family history of breast cancer but not ovarian cancer were followed in a recently published study from Memorial Sloan-Kettering Cancer Center and were not found to have an increased incidence of ovarian cancer.

94. Should I have genetic counseling? How do you determine who should go for genetic testing?

If you have a family history of ovarian or breast cancer (or both) you're at increased risk of ovarian cancer. For you, genetic counseling makes sense, especially if you have sisters or young children and you're worried that they may have inherited a gene mutation. In addition, if you have a strong family history of multiple types of cancers, getting genetic counseling may make sense.

If you have two first-degree (immediate family) relatives (i.e., mother and sister) affected with ovarian or breast cancer, your probability of having a genetic mutation increases dramatically. The same is true if you or a first-degree relative have had both breast and ovarian cancer. A family history of colon cancer or colon polyps and ovarian cancer also raises your possibility of having a gene mutation. Finally, if your extended family history includes multiple affected members with varying types of cancer, including ovarian cancer, you may want to obtain genetic testing. If you are still unsure, it's always worthwhile to discuss genetic counseling with your doctor.

Unfortunately, being told that you have a genetic mutation associated with a cancer risk is often a double-edged sword. It may raise issues within yourself or your family as to what can be done about this risk. Should you have your breasts removed to prevent breast cancer? If you don't have ovarian cancer, should you have your ovaries removed? These surgeries when done to prevent cancer are termed prophylactic procedures. Working through such issues is difficult and makes a genetic counselor all the more important so that you can fully understand the risk of cancer in your specific situation and the potential pros and cons of prophylactic surgery.

Notably, recently published reports suggest that prophylactically removing the ovaries in women who have BRCA mutations may decrease the risk of future breast or ovarian cancer.

Dee's comments:

When I was first diagnosed, I did not realize that there was a hereditary link for ovarian cancer and breast cancer. Both my sister and maternal aunt had been diagnosed with breast cancer, my sister at the age of 42. Because of that knowledge, I was very diligent regarding annual mammograms and visits to my gynecologist. Ovarian cancer was not even on my radar.

After my diagnosis, I talked to the genetics counselor at Rutgers Cancer Institute of New Jersey and my gynecologic oncologist. After reviewing my family history, the genetics counselor recommended that I have the genetic testing. I agreed because I had learned that genetic information could impact my treatment plan, as well as guide my daughter's health care and surveillance.

95. Is there any way to screen for ovarian cancer?

The quick answer to this question is that there are no worthwhile screening tests for ovarian cancer for the general population. The worth of a screening program depends on three factors: the sensitivity of the test, which is the probability that a test result will be positive in a person with the disease, called the **true positive rate**; the specificity of the test, or the probability of a negative test result in a patient without the disease, called the **true negative rate**; and the prevalence of the disease, or the number of cases seen in a year. These three factors will determine the predictive value of the test.

Some physicians use annual CA-125 tests and transvaginal ultrasound to look for signs of cancer in women known to be at risk. However, neither of these tests is based on good evidence, only on expert opinion. Although its accuracy has been established, the sensitivity of transvaginal ultrasound has to be taken in the context of the incidence of ovarian cancer, which is low in the general population. Thus, the predictive value of a positive ultrasound is less than 10% and increases to only 27% if combined with an elevated CA-125 result. Furthermore, screening for ovarian cancer has not been shown to result in a decrease in the mortality rate from the disease, and there remains a high risk of false-positive results. However, the work on screening remains an area of very active investigation.

Thus, researchers have not recommended screening in the general population. Current research is focusing on the value of screening in a group of women considered to be at high risk for ovarian cancer and on other mechanisms of early detection, including the use of novel

PREVENTION, SCREENING, AND ADVOCACY

True positive rate

The proportion of patients who have a positive test result and who do have the disease.

True negative rate

The proportion of patients who have a negative test result and who do not have the disease.

serum markers or the use of proteomics. All that being said, for a woman at high risk, serial CA-125 and ultrasound every 6 months are commonly performed, but the benefit of this strategy still remains to be seen.

96. What kind of research is being conducted to cure this cancer?

The research being conducted in this field is extensive. Major efforts are under way to improve the early detection of this cancer so that we may pick it up when it hasn't spread and hence it can more likely be cured. Some of this work is exploring novel markers that may one day replace the CA-125 test as a more reliable and earlier indicator of ovarian cancer. Others are exploring the newer technologies of gene profiling (**genomics**) and protein profiling (**proteomics**) that may tip off doctors to the presence of cancer, even before it can show up on imaging tests.

Genomics

The study of gene expression patterns.

Proteomics

The study of protein profiles.

Work is also being done to improve surgery for ovarian cancer. Gynecological oncologists are leaders in laparoscopic surgery which may one day be an option for surgical staging (discussed in Question 18 on page 30). Others are looking into more aggressive surgical operations that could obtain a higher number of women whose tumors can be optimally resected.

In addition, we are aiming to learn more about the genetics and the biology of ovarian cancer. Through work done with samples as part of the Cancer Genome Atlas, we are learning that ovarian cancer is not one disease, but multiple different types. For example, serous ovarian cancers appear to have a genetic make-up more similar to aggressive breast and uterine cancers, than to other histologic types of ovarian cancer. This work will hopefully help us find molecular targets that we can exploit for treatment, and will help push the aim of a more personalized (or precise) approach to treatment.

One day, we hope to be able to use a pill that will specifically target the cancer and not the surrounding tissue; our hope is to make the delivery (administration) of medical therapy more convenient and, more importantly, to reduce its side effects and toxicity.

Finally, researchers continue to explore ways to enable the immune system to recognize the cancer cell as foreign, so that it can kill cancer by itself. Investigators recently showed that the presence of immune cells (**T-cells**) in the cancer points to a better prognosis for patients than that obtained from tumors without T-cells. This finding supports the hypothesis that the immune system plays a role in trying to defeat or contain cancer and points to another mode of treatment that can be explored.

T-cells

Immune cells that primarily fight viruses. They are being used in clinical trials of immunotherapy for ovarian and other cancers.

97. Should I research and learn more about the disease and its treatment?

When you are diagnosed with ovarian cancer, you may find yourself becoming an advocate by default—your own advocate! Indeed, it is our hope that you are reading this book because you want to know how to be proactive in your own care. When it comes to ovarian cancer, it is useful to know what you are faced with, and that is part of why this book was written. But it also helps for you to be aggressive about gathering information and asking questions. So our immediate answer to this question would be, yes, you should learn more, but do so at your own pace. Don't feel you need to become an expert overnight. Remember, too, that your emotions about your diagnosis should not be shunted aside as you pursue your ovarian cancer education. Take it slowly enough that you can absorb the information and grow comfortable with it before you continue.

As you grow more knowledgeable and become closely involved in your treatment, you may also find yourself becoming an advocate for others. Perhaps you will join a support group and offer support, advice, or just a badly needed ear for someone who needs to talk. Just as teachers learn their subject better through teaching, this sort of advocacy can help you as well as help others. If you want to take it a step further, consider volunteering for an advocacy organization such as those listed in the **Additional Resources**, where you can work to raise awareness of the disease or lobby for funding in support of research. If you have the energy and the inclination for this activity, it can prove helpful not only to ovarian cancer patients in general, but also to you specifically. For instance, you would be in a position to know of advances in treatment when they first become available, rather than waiting for your doctor to hear of them and recommend them to you. Again, this depends on how you as an individual feel about these activities; public advocacy is not for everyone, no matter what its advantages.

Whatever road you take, be it personal education or public advocacy, be aware of one drawback: There is so much information and so much data out there that it is not uncommon for women to get lost in the statistics. It is all too easy to forget that statistics are generalizations about ovarian cancer that, like most statistics, are so broad they are meaningless for an individual. Take them too seriously, and you may find them overwhelming. Try to find methods that will work for you without making you anxious or depressed about your disease.

Dee's comments:

I have often described myself as a research "hound." The scientist in me (I have degrees in biochemical engineering and material science) really likes to read research journals and learn as much as I can about the disease, genetics, and treatments.

In doing this research, I have learned that there are some unreliable sources on the Internet. Many times, misinformation is what is shared quickly online and is difficult to refute. I use government sources (NCI, CDC), medical organizations (ASCO, SGO, ACS), reviewed journals, and the websites of comprehensive cancer centers when I look up information online.

98. Where can I get support?

You can consider a cancer diagnosis sort of like an invitation to join an exclusive women's club that you never expected or desired to join. This is an important concept because it relays a very important message: You are not alone. An entire community of women live with and fight this cancer; they are in a situation similar to yours, no matter where you are along the cancer path; and they are available to you for advice, support, or just helping with the day-to-day struggles of life with cancer. In addition, support groups are available in most local communities. We who treat cancer know that this is a disease that has an impact not only on a patient, but also on everyone who cares about her and loves her. Your nurses are often the best source of information, and they should be able to direct you toward these support groups locally or to a therapist, in case you need to talk things out in a safe and private environment. As cancer care providers, we're here not only to help you manage your cancer, but also to help you deal with the fear and questions that accompany it.

99. When should I ask for help?

Being diagnosed with ovarian cancer is an incredibly scary process, and no one should go through it alone. If you're feeling isolated and scared, you should reach out for support. Sadness and anxiety are common in women who have just been told that they have cancer. Most women tell me that they feel it's a death sentence and only remember what they read about Gilda Radner's brave but short struggle with this cancer. If you don't discuss them, the fears can build and make the work that must be done too hard. They can also cause a worsening sense that you're alone, and that feeds into a cycle of deepening despair. If this describes what you or someone you love is going through, reach out for help.

Such feelings must be brought out into the open. Anyone diagnosed with ovarian cancer must want to fight it and must trust that treatments are available and successful and can give you back your life. Even if the cancer comes back, there's reason to be hopeful. As discussed in Question 71, distress is common and can be debilitating, but it does not have to be. Palliative care can be a source of information and support as you are treated for and live through, and then beyond, ovarian cancer. No one should wait until they are told they are dying to access palliative care—it is much more than that, and can bring many more benefits, earlier on than at the end of life.

Sometimes, antidepressant and antianxiety medications are necessary to help you to come to grips with a cancer diagnosis and the change it requires in your life. Medications to help you handle the diagnosis, its challenges, and treatment are not signs of weakness. There are resources available to enable you to regain control of your life so that you can handle the decisions important to fighting this disease.

100. Where can I get more information?

Many resources are available for women newly diagnosed or living with a diagnosis of ovarian cancer. These include the organizations, Web sites, and books listed on the following pages. Many more resources are available besides those listed here; check your local library or Amazon.com for books, or go to any of the following organizations' Web sites and search for links or resources related to ovarian cancer.

Additional Resources

Organizations

American Cancer Society
1599 Clifton Road
Atlanta, GA 30329
Phone: 800-ACS-2345
Website: www.cancer.org

American Society of Clinical Oncology
1900 Duke Street, Suite 200
Alexandria, VA 22314
Phone: 703-299-0150
Websites: www.asco.org
            www.cancer.net (ASCO's patient education website)

Cancer Care, Inc.
275 Seventh Avenue
Floor 22
New York, NY 10001
Phone: 800-813-4673
Website: www.cancercare.org

Cancer Research Institute
One Exchange Plaza
55 Broadway, Suite 1802
New York, NY 10006
Phone: 800-99-CANCER (800-992-2623)
Website: www.cancerresearch.org

Centers for Disease Control and Prevention
1600 Clifton Road
Atlanta, GA 30333
Phone: 404-639-3534
Toll-free: 800-311-3435
Website: www.cdc.gov

Department of Veterans Affairs
Veterans Health Association
810 Vermont Avenue, N.W.
Washington, DC 20420
Phone: 202-273-5400 (Washington, DC office)
Toll-free: 800-827-1000 (Local VA office)
Website: www.va.gov

Foundation for Women's Cancer
230 W. Monroe Suite 2528
Chicago, IL 60606-4902
Phone: 312-578-1439
Fax: 312-578-9769
Website: www.foundationforwomenscancer.org

Gilda's Club (New York City)
195 West Houston Street
New York, NY 10014
Phone: 212-647-9700
Fax: 212-647-1151
Website: http://www.gildasclubnyc.org

Health Resources and Services Administration—Hill-Burton Program
U.S. Department of Health and Human Services
Parklawn Building
5600 Fishers Lane
Rockville, MD 20857
Phone: 301-443-5656
Toll-free: 800-638-0742/800-492-0359
   (From the Maryland area)
Website: www.hrsa.gov/about/index.html

Institute of Certified Financial Planners
Phone: 303-759-4900
Toll-free: 800-282-7526 (Automated referral service)
Website: www.icfp.org

LiveStrong
2201 E. Sixth Street
Austin, Texas 78702
Phone: 855.220.7777
Websites: http://www.livestrong.org
http://www.livestrong.com/

National Cancer Institute
National Cancer Institute Public Information Office
Building 31, Room 10A31
31 Center Drive, MSC 2580
Bethesda, MD 20892-2580
Phone: 301-435-3848 (Public Information Office line)
Website: www.cancer.gov

National Center for Complementary and Alternative Medicine
NCCAM Clearinghouse
P.O. Box 7923
Gaithersburg, MD 20898
Phone: 888-644-6226
Website: www.nccam.nih.gov

National Comprehensive Cancer Network
50 Huntingdon Pike, Suite 200
Rockledge, PA 19046
Phone: 888-909-NCCN (888-909-6226)
Website: www.nccn.org

National Ovarian Cancer Coalition
500 NE Spanish River Boulevard, Suite 14
Boca Raton, FL 33431
Phone: 561-393-0005
Toll-free: 888-OVARIAN
Fax: 561-393-7275
Website: www.ovarian.org

National Viatical Association of America
1200 19th Street, N.W.
Washington, DC 20036-2412
Phone: 202-429-5129
Toll-free: 800-741-9465
Website: www.nationalviatical.org

National Women's Health Information Center
U.S. Department of Health and Human Services
8550 Arlington Boulevard, Suite 300
Fairfax, VA 22031
Phone: 800-994-9662
Website: www.womenshealth.gov

Office of Minority Health
U.S. Department of Health and Human Services
P.O. Box 37337
Washington, DC 20013-7337
Phone: 800-444-6472
Website: minorityhealth.hhs.gov

Ovarian Cancer National Alliance
910 17th Street, N.W., Suite 1190
Washington, DC 20006
Phone: 202-331-1332
Fax: 202-331-2292
Website: www.ovariancancer.org

SHARE
1501 Broadway, Suite 704A
New York, NY 10036
Phone: 212-719-1204 or toll-free: 866-537-4273
Website: www.sharecancersupport.org

Sharsheret
1086 Teaneck Road, Suite 2G
Teaneck, New Jersey 07666
Phone: 866.474.2774
Website: http://www.sharsheret.org/

A resource for the Jewish community facing breast and ovarian cancer

Social Security Administration
Office of Public Inquiries
6401 Security Boulevard., Room 4-C-5 Annex
Baltimore, MD 21235-6401
Toll-free: 800-772-1213 or 800-325-0778 (TTY)
Website: www.ssa.gov

Society of Gynecologic Oncologists
401 N. Michigan Avenue
Chicago, IL 60611
Phone: 312-644-6610
Website: www.sgo.org

United Seniors Health Cooperative
409 3rd Street, S.W., Suite 200
Washington, DC 20024
Phone: 202-479-6973
Toll-free: 800-637-2604
Website: www.unitedseniorshealth.org

Online Resources

CancerLinks (www.cancerlinks.org)

CancerNet (http://cancernet.nci.nih.gov)
    Detailed information provided by the National
    Cancer Institute on many types of cancer.

CancerSource (www.cancersource.com)

Eyes on the Prize (www.eyesontheprize.org)
    A support community for women living with gyne-
    cologic cancer.

Women's Cancer Network (www.wcn.org)

Caregivers and Home Care

Association of Cancer Online Resources
Website: www.acor.org

Click on "Mailing Lists" and then select "Caregivers
& Family Issues" for an online discussion group for
caregivers of cancer patients.

**Caring for the Caregiver (National Coalition for
Cancer Survivorship)**
Website: www.canceradvocacy.org/resources
    /cancer-survival-toolbox/special-topics
    /caring-for-the-caregiver/

Family Caregiver Alliance
690 Market Street, Suite 600
San Francisco, CA 94104
Phone: 415-434-3388
Website: www.caregiver.org

Caregiver resources include an online support group and an information clearinghouse. Information available in Spanish.

Guide for Cancer Supporters: Step-by-Step Ways to Help a Relative or Friend Fight Cancer (R.A. Bloch Cancer Foundation)
Website: www.blochcancer.org.

Click on "Info For Supporters."

National Family Caregivers Association
10400 Connecticut Avenue, #500
Kensington, MD 20895-3944
Phone: 800-896-3650
Website: www.nfcacares.org

Provides education, information, support, and advocacy services for family caregivers.

Children

Kids Konnected
27071 Cabot Road, Suite 102
Laguna Hills, CA 92653
Phone: 949-582-5443
Website: www.kidskonnected.org

Provides extensive support resources and programs for children who have a parent with cancer.

What Do I Tell the Children?—A Guide for a Parent with Cancer (Cancerbackup)

Web page: www.cancerbackup.org.uk/info /talk-children.htm

Clinical Trials Resources

There is no single resource for locating clinical trials for ovarian cancer. It makes sense to check all of the resources listed below repeatedly because new trials are continually added. There are also clinical trials services emerging that help to match patients to clinical trials. Some of these services can be useful for obtaining information and saving time, but it is important to read the company's privacy statement and be aware of whether the company is being paid for recruiting patients.

National Cancer Institute Clinical Trials

Phone: 800-4CANCER

Website: www.cancer.gov/clinicaltrials

The NCI offers comprehensive information on understanding and finding clinical trials, including access to the NCI/PDQ Clinical Trials Database.

National Institutes of Health/National Library of Medicine Clinical Trials

Website: ClinicalTrials.gov

Clinical trials database service developed by the National Institute of Health's National Library of Medicine.

Centerwatch Clinical Trials Listing Service

Website: www.centerwatch.com

Listing of clinical trials conducted by drug companies.

NCI Clinical Trials and Insurance Coverage

Web page: http://www.cancer.gov/clinicaltrials
/learningabout/payingfor

Excellent in-depth guide to clinical trials insurance issues.

Complementary and Alternative Medicine (CAM)

American Academy of Medical Acupuncture

Website: www.medicalacupuncture.org

Professional site with articles on acupuncture, a list of frequently asked questions, and an acupuncturist locator.

Commonweal

P.O. Box 316

Bolinas, CA 94924

Phone: 415-868-0970

Website: www.commonweal.org

Provides information on complementary approaches to cancer care, including the full text of Michael Lerner's 1994 book, *Choices in Healing: Integrating the Best of Conventional and Complementary Approaches to Cancer*, published by MIT press (updated version available in print).

National Center for Complementary and Alternative Medicine (NCCAM)

Website: http://nccam.nih.gov

Offers information on complementary and alternative medicine therapies, including NCI/PDQ expert-reviewed fact sheets on individual therapies and dietary supplements.

NCI Office of Cancer Complementary and Alternative Medicine (OCCAM)

Website: www.cancer.gov/occam

Information clearinghouse supporting the NCI's CAM activities.

Diet and Nutrition

American Institute for Cancer Research

1759 R Street, N.W.
Washington, DC 20009
Phone: 800-843-8114 or 202-328-7744 (in DC)
Website: www.aicr.org

Supports research on diet and nutrition in the prevention and treatment of cancer. Provides information to cancer patients on nutrition and cancer, including a compilation of healthy recipes. Maintains a nutrition hotline for questions relating to nutrition and health.

Nutrition (American Cancer Society)

Website: www.cancer.org. Enter "nutrition" in the search box.

Nutrition resources include: ACS guidelines on nutrition, dietary supplement information, nutrition message boards, and tips on low-fat cooking and choosing healthy ingredients.

Drugs/Medications

MedlinePlus: Drug Information
Website: www.medlineplus.gov. Click on "Drugs & Supplements."

A guide to over 9,000 prescription and over-the-counter medications provided by U.S. Pharmacopeia (USP).

Employment, Insurance, Financial, and Legal Resources

ORGANIZATIONS AND PROGRAMS

Americans with Disabilities Act (U.S. Department of Justice)
Cancer Legal Resource Center
919 S. Albany Street
Los Angeles, CA 90019-10015
Phone: 213-736-1455
Website: www.usdoj.gov/crt/ada/adahom1.htm

A joint program of Loyola Law School and the Western Law Center for Disability Rights. Provides information and educational outreach on cancer-related legal issues to people with cancer and others impacted by the disease.

America's Health Insurance Plans (AHIP)
601 Pennsylvania Avenue, NW South Building, Suite 500
Washington, DC 20004
Website: www.hiaa.org
Phone: 800-509-4422

Provides insurance guides for consumers. Topics include health insurance and managed care, disability income, long-term care, and medical savings accounts.

Centers for Medicare & Medicaid Services (CMS)
(formerly the Health Care Financing Administration [HCFA])
Website: www.cms.hhs.gov

Oversees administration of:
- Medicare—Federal health insurance program for people 65 years or older and some disabled people under 65 years of age.
  Phone: 800-633-4227
  Website: www.medicare.gov
- Medicaid—Federal–state health insurance program for certain low-income people. Contact your state Medicaid offices for further information.
  Website: www.cms.hhs.gov/home/medicaid.asp
- Health Insurance Portability and Accountability Act (HIPAA)—Insurance reform that may lower your chance of losing existing coverage, ease your ability to switch health plans, and/or help you buy coverage on your own if you lose your employer's plan and have no other coverage available.
  Website: www.cms.hhs.gov/HIPAAGenInfo/

Family and Medical Leave Act (FMLA)
Website: http://www.dol.gov/whd/fmla/

Hill-Burton Program (Health Resources and Services Administration)
Phone: 301-443-5656
Toll-free: 800-638-0742 (800-492-0359 in Maryland)
Website: http://www.hrsa.gov/gethealthcare
  /affordable/hillburton/

Facilities that receive Hill-Burton funds from the government are required by law to provide services to some people who cannot afford to pay. Information on Hill-Burton eligibility and facilities locations is available via phone or the Internet.

Patient Advocate Foundation

421 Butler Farm Road
Hampton, VA 23666
Phone: 800-532-5274
Fax: 757-873-8999
Website: www.patientadvocate.org

Nonprofit organization helps patients to resolve insurance, debt, and job discrimination matters relative to cancer. Patient resources include *The National Financial Resources Guidebook for Patients: A State-by-State Directory, Your Guide to the Appeals Process,* and the *Managed Care Answer Guide.*

Social Security Administration (SSA)

Website: www.ssa.gov

Oversees two programs that pay benefits to people with disabilities:
- Social Security Disability Insurance—Pays benefits to you and certain members of your family if you have worked long enough and paid Social Security taxes.
- Supplemental Security Income—Supplements Social Security payments based on need.

Veterans Health Administration

810 Vermont Avenue, N.W.
Washington, DC 20420
Phone: Benefits: 1-800-827-1000
         Health Care: 1-877-222-VETS (8387)
Website: www.va.gov/health/

Eligible veterans and their dependents may receive cancer treatment at a Veterans Administration Medical Center.

FINANCIAL ASSISTANCE PROGRAMS

Air Care Alliance
Phone: 888-260-9707
Website: www.aircareall.org

Network of organizations willing to provide public benefit flights for health care.

Finding Ways to Pay for Care (National Coalition for Cancer Survivorship)
Website: www.cansearch.org. Select "Programs" and then "Cancer Survival Toolbox."

NeedyMeds
Website: www.needymeds.com

Information on patient assistance programs and other programs that help people obtain medications, supplies, and equipment.

Hospice and End-of-Life Issues

Partnership for Caring
1620 Eye Street, N.W., Suite 202
Washington, DC 20006
Phone: 202-296-8071
Toll-free: 800-989-9455
Website: www.partnershipforcaring.org

Comprehensive information and resources covering end-of-life issues, including advance directives.

Association of Online Cancer Resources, Cancer-Hospice mailing list

Website: www.acor.org. Click on "Mailing Lists," select "Hospice," and then select "Cancer-Hospice."

Online discussion group for cancer patients dealing with hospice issues.

Growth House

Website: www.growthhouse.org

Extensive, annotated directory of hospice and end-of-life resources organized by topic.

Home Care Guide for Advanced Cancer (American College of Physicians)

Website: www.acponline.org/public/h_care/

Guide for family and friends caring for advanced cancer patients who are living at home.

Hospice Net

Website: www.hospicenet.org

Provides comprehensive information to patients and families facing life-threatening illness. Extensive resources addressing end-of-life issues from both patient and caregiver perspectives.

Patient Advocacy Skills

Cancer Survival Toolbox (National Coalition for Cancer Survivorship)

Website: www.cansearch.org. Select "Programs" and then "Cancer Survival Toolbox."

Topics include communication skills, finding information, solving problems, making decisions, negotiating, and standing up for your rights. (Also available as audiotapes at 877-866-5748.)

Physician and Hospital Locators

American Society of Clinical Oncology (ASCO)
Website: www.asco.org. Click on the "Find an Oncologist" button.

American College of Surgeons (ACS) Commission on Cancer
Website: www.facs.org/cpm/default.htm

Listing of ACS Commission on Cancer's Approved Hospital Cancer Programs.

American Medical Association (AMA) DoctorFinder
Website: www.ama-assn.org/aps/amahg.htm

Provides professional information on licensed U.S. physicians.

Prevention and Risk Assessment

Prevention (American Cancer Society)
Website: www.cancer.org. Enter "prevention" in the search box.

Comprehensive section on prevention covers topics such as environmental and occupational cancer risks, exercise, tobacco and cancer, nutrition for risk reduction, and prevention and detection programs.

Research Resources and Reference

**PubMed: MEDLINE
(National Library of Medicine)**
Website: www.ncbi.nlm.nih.gov/PubMed/

Provides free online access to MEDLINE, a database of over 11 million citations to the medical literature.

Medscape

Website: www.medscape.com. Enter "ovarian cancer" in the search box.

Medscape is an excellent source for the latest news in lung cancer research, including access to summaries of cancer conferences. The site is aimed at health care professionals. Registration is required for free access to Medscape.

Support Services

Association of Cancer Online Resources (ACOR)

Website: www.acor.org. Click on "Mailing Lists."

ACOR offers online support groups for cancer patients.

Cancer Care

275 Seventh Avenue
New York, NY 10001
Phone: 212-712-8080
Toll-free: 800-813-4673
Website: www.cancercare.org

Provides comprehensive support services and programs to people with cancer.

Cancer Survivors Network

Website: www.acscsn.org

The Cancer Survivors Network is the American Cancer Society's online patient community.

R.A. Bloch Cancer Foundation
4400 Main Street
Kansas City, MO 64111
Phone: 816-932-8453
Toll-free: 800-433-0464
Website: www.blochcancer.org

Provides Bloch-authored cancer books free of charge, a multidisciplinary referral service, and patient-to-patient phone support.

Vital Options International
15060 Ventura Boulevard, Suite 211
Sherman Oaks, CA 91403
Phone: 818-788-5225
Website: www.vitaloptions.org

Produces "The Group Room," a weekly, syndicated radio call-in show (with simultaneous Webcast) covering important and timely topics in cancer.

Wellness Community
35 East Seventh Street, Suite 412
Cincinnati, OH 45202
Phone: 513-421-7111
Toll-free: 888-793-WELL
Website: www.wellness-community.org

Provides educational programs and support groups for people with cancer and their families.

Talking About Cancer (American Cancer Society)
Website: www.cancer.org. Enter "Talking About Cancer" in the search box.

Discusses how to talk about your cancer with family, friends, your health care providers, and your employer. Includes resources for locating in-person and online support groups.

Coping with Cancer
Phone: 615-791-3859
Website: www.copingmag.com

Cancer magazine available free of charge in oncology offices or by subscription.

Symptoms, Side Effects, and Complications

FATIGUE

CancerFatigue.org
Website: www.cancerfatigue.org

Information about cancer-related fatigue for patients and caregivers.

Association of Cancer Online Resources Cancer-Fatigue mailing list
Website: www.acor.org. Click on "Mailing Lists," select "C," and then select "Cancer-Fatigue."

Online discussion list covering cancer and treatment-related fatigue.

National Comprehensive Cancer Network Cancer-Related Fatigue and Anemia Treatment Guidelines for Patients
Website: www.nccn.org/patients/patient_gls
   /_english/_fatigue/contents.asp

NAUSEA AND VOMITING

National Comprehensive Cancer Network Nausea and Vomiting Treatment Guidelines for Patients with Cancer

Web page: www.nccn.org/patient_gls/_english
/_nausea_and_vomiting/contents.asp

NCI/PDQ Nausea and Vomiting

Website: www.cancer.gov Enter "nausea" in the search box.

Expert-reviewed information summary about cancer-related nausea and vomiting.

NUTRITIONAL PROBLEMS

NCI/PDQ Nutrition

Website: www.cancer.gov. Enter "nutrition" in the search box.

Expert-reviewed information summary about the causes and management of nutritional problems occurring in cancer patients.

PAIN

The National Pain Foundation (NPF)

P.O. Box 102605
Denver, CO 80250-2605
Website: www.NationalPainFoundation.org

The NPF Website offers online education and support communities for pain patients and their families, including cancer pain and palliative care resources.

Association of Cancer Online Resources Cancer Pain mailing list
Website: www.acor.org. Click on "Mailing Lists," select "C," and then select "Cancer-Pain."

Online discussion list about pain associated with cancer and its treatments.

NCCN Cancer Pain Treatment Guidelines for Patients
Website: www.nccn.org/patients/patient_gls
/_english/_pain/contents.asp

NCI/PDQ Pain
Website: www.cancer.gov. Enter "pain" in the search box.

Expert-reviewed information summary about cancer-related pain. Includes discussion of approaches to the management and treatment of cancer-associated pain.

PERIPHERAL NEUROPATHY

The Neuropathy Association
60 East 42nd Street, Suite 942
New York, NY 10165
Phone: 212-692-0662
Website: www.neuropathy.org

Association of Cancer Online Resources Cancer-Neuropathy mailing list
Website: www.acor.org Click on "Mailing Lists," click on "C," and then select "Cancer-Neuropathy."

Online discussion group for patients dealing with neuropathy induced by cancer or its treatments.

Almadrones, L.A., & Arcot, R. Patient Guide to Peripheral Neuropathy. *Oncology Nursing Forum.* 1999;26(8):1359–1362.

PLEURAL EFFUSION

Chemical Pleurodesis for Malignant Pleural Effusion (Cancer Supportive Care)

Website: www.cancersupportivecare.com
/pleural.html

Carolyn Clary-Macy, RN, provides a clear explanation of chemical pleurodesis for malignant pleural effusion. Aimed at patients.

SEXUAL EFFECTS

Association of Cancer Online Resources Cancer-Fertility and Cancer-Sexuality mailing lists

Website: www.acor.org. Click on "Mailing Lists," select "C," and then select "Cancer-Fertility" and/or "Cancer-Sexuality."

Online discussion lists about fertility and sexuality issues associated with cancer.

NCI/PDQ Sexuality and Reproductive Issues

Website: www.cancer.gov. Enter "sexuality" in the search box.

Expert-reviewed information summary about factors that may affect fertility and sexual functioning in people who have cancer.

Tests and Procedures

Diagnostic Imaging (MEDLINEplus)

Website: www.nlm.nih.gov/medlineplus
/diagnosticimaging.html

Laboratory Tests (MEDLINEplus)
Website: www.nlm.nih.gov/medlineplus
/laboratorytests.html

Margolis, Simeon, ed. *The Johns Hopkins Consumer Guide to Medical Tests: What You Can Expect, How You Should Prepare, What Your Results Mean.* Baltimore, MD: The Johns Hopkins University Press, 2001.

Treatment Information and Guidelines

Chemotherapy and You (NIH/NCI)
Website: www.cancer.gov. Enter "Chemotherapy and You" in the search box. Also available in print by calling 800-4CANCER.

Radiation Therapy and You (NIH/NCI)
Website: www.cancer.gov. Enter "Radiation Therapy and You" in the search box. Also available in print by calling 800-4CANCER.

Survivorship Issues

Association of Cancer Online Resources
LT-Survivors mailing list
Website: www.acor.org. Click on "Mailing Lists," select "L," and then select "LT-SURVIVORS."

Forum for discussion of issues of concern to long-term cancer survivors.

Books and Pamphlets

The following books are available from the American Cancer Society:

- *American Cancer Society's Guide to Complementary and Alternative Cancer Methods*
- *The American Cancer Society's Guide to Pain Control: Powerful Methods to Overcome Cancer Pain*
- *Coming to Terms with Cancer*
- *Informed Decisions*, 2nd Edition

The following pamphlets are available from the National Cancer Institute:

- *Chemotherapy and You: A Guide to Self-Help During Treatment*
- *Eating Hints for Cancer Patients Before, During, and After Treatment*
- *Helping Yourself During Chemotherapy*
- *Taking Part in Clinical Trials: What Cancer Patients Need to Know*
- *Taking Time: Support for People with Cancer and the People Who Care About Them*

Available in Spanish:

- *En que consisten los estudios clinicos? Un folleto para los pacientes de cancer*

The following pamphlets are available from the National Comprehensive Cancer Network:

- Available in Spanish: *El dolor asociado con el cáncer*

Available from The Wellness Community:

- *A Patient Active Guide to Living With Ovarian Cancer*

BOOKS AND ARTICLES

Benigno, B.B. *The Ultimate Guide to Ovarian Cancer.* Atlanta, GA: Sherryben Publishing House, LLC, 2013.

Bloch, A.S., Grant, B., Hamilton, K.K., & Thomson, C.A., eds. *American Cancer Society Complete Guide to Nutrition for Cancer Survivors: Eating Well, Staying Well During and After Cancer.* Atlanta, GA: American Cancer Society, 2010.

Coggins, J.M. *Ovarian Cancer? You CanNOT be serious!* Bloomington, IN: AuthorHouse, 2013.

Conner, K., & Langford, L. *Ovarian Cancer: Your Guide to Taking Control.* Sebastopol, CA: O'Reilly Media/Patient Centered Guides, 2003.

Dizon, D.S., & Campos, S.M. *Dx/Rx Gynecologic Cancer.* Sudbury, MA: Jones & Bartlett Learning, 2010.

Friedman, S., Sutphen, R., & Steligo, K. *Confronting Hereditary Breast and Ovarian Cancer: Identify Your Risk, Understand your Options, Change Your Destiny.* Baltimore, MD: Johns Hopkins University Press, 2012.

Gubar, S. *Memoir of a Debulked Woman: Enduring Ovarian Cancer.* New York: WW Norton and Company, 2013.

Ingalis, K., & Wiechmann. A. *Outshine: An Ovarian Cancer Memoir.* Edina, MN: Beaver's Pond Press, 2014.

Katz, A. *Women Cancer Sex.* Fullerton, CA: Hygeia Media, 2009.

Krychman, M.L. *100 Questions & Answers for Women Living With Cancer: A Practical Guide for Survivorship.* Sudbury, MA: Jones & Bartlett Learning, 2007.

Levine, D.A., Dizon, D.S., Yasher, C.M., et al. *Handbook for Principles and Practice of Gynecologic Oncology*, 2nd ed. Philadelphia: Lippincott Williams & Wilkins, 2015.

Miron, A. *Ovarian Cancer Journeys: Survivors Share Their Stories To Help Others.* iUniverse, Inc., 2004.

Montz, F.J., & Bristow, R.E. *A Guide to Survivorship for Women with Ovarian Cancer.* Baltimore, MD: Johns Hopkins University Press, 2005.

Salani, R., & Bristow, R. *Johns Hopkins Patients' Guide to Ovarian Cancer.* Sudbury, MA: Jones & Bartlett Learning, 2009.

Tewari, K., & Monk, B. *The 21st Century Handbook of Clinical Ovarian Cancer.* Auckland, NZ: Adis International, 2015.

GLOSSARY

A

Adenocarcinomas: Type of cancer, arising from the cells of epithelial origin.

Adenomas: Noncancerous tumors arising from epithelial cells.

Adjuvant: Given after a primary procedure.

Anechoic: Used in ultrasound studies, describes a lack of different ultrasound signals, commonly seen with simple cysts.

Angiogenesis inhibitors: Drugs that block the formation of new blood vessels.

Antiangiogenesis: To block new blood vessel formation.

Antigen: A protein that sits on or is released from cells that can be targeted with an antibody or a vaccine.

Antihistamine: To block the release of histamines, which are often associated with allergic reactions.

Apoptosis: Programmed cell death.

Ascites: Fluid build-up within the abdomen.

Atypia: Used by pathologists, it describes abnormal cellular changes seen under the microscope.

B

Belly wash: Common term for an intraperitoneal treatment.

Benign: Not cancerous.

Bilateral salpingo-oophorectomy: The surgical term for removal of both the right and left fallopian tubes and ovaries.

Biopsy: Removal of a small amount of tissue for analysis by a pathologist. It can be done during surgery or before surgery using other less invasive procedures.

Borderline: A term used to describe a tumor that does not appear normal but does not meet a pathologist's criteria for cancer; otherwise described as low malignant potential.

Bowel obstruction: Condition where the small or large bowel is blocked due to either adhesions or tumor that causes the bowel to back up instead of work normally (to get rid of stool).

Bowel perforation: A rupture of the bowel wall.

C

Capillaries: The smallest blood vessels within your body.

Carcinomatosis: Cancer deposits along the abdomen, often along the bowel and involving the omentum.

Colon: The large intestine, part of your gastrointestinal tract. Its function is to absorb water and food and to excrete stool.

Colonic dilation: Swelling of the bowel due to gas or liquid that cannot move through.

Colostomy: A loop of bowel that is pulled through your skin.

Complete resection: Removal of all the tumor in your abdomen and pelvis.

Computed tomography: Otherwise known as a CT scan, this is a highly sensitive radiology exam used to help diagnose and follow patients with cancer.

Cremaphore: A molecule to which drugs are attached to increase the drugs' delivery into your body.

Cytology: The process of examining cells under the microscope; the sample is usually obtained from floating cells in the fluid of the abdomen (ascites) or chest (pleural effusions).

D

Differentiation: The process of cells maturing so they can perform specific processes in our bodies.

Direct extension: The process by which cancer extends into local and surrounding tissue.

Dyspepsia: Pain in the stomach.

Dyspnea: Shortness of breath.

E

Early satiety: Feeling of getting full faster than you normally would.

Echogenic: An ultrasound term describing complex patterns seen within a cyst.

Endodermal sinus tumor: A type of germ-cell tumor, derived from early cells destined to become eggs. Otherwise, they are referred to as yolk-sac tumors.

Endoscopic camera: A flexible camera within a tube (the endoscope) that is used to do minimally invasive procedures.

Erythropoietin: A hormone produced by the kidneys to stimulate the release of red blood cells in the bone marrow.

Estrogen: A female hormone produced by the ovaries; it is responsible for female changes during maturity.

F

First-degree relatives: Blood relatives of your immediate family (father, mother, sister, or brother).

Fistulas: Abnormally formed channels between two otherwise separate organs, such as between the vagina and bladder (vesicovaginal) or between the bowel and the skin (enterocutaneous).

Founder Effect: Greater inheritance of a genetic mutation in a well-defined population that can theoretically be traced back to a common ancestor.

G

Gastroenterologist: A medical specialist in treating disorders of the esophagus, stomach, bowel, and rectum.

Genomics: The study of gene expression patterns.

Grade: A pathologist term that defines how abnormal a cell is under the microscope.

Gynecological oncologist: A specialist in the treatment of cancer of the female reproductive system.

H

Hematogenous dissemination: A process of spreading by which cancer travels through the bloodstream.

Hydronephrosis: Abnormal enlargement of the kidney.

Hydroureteronephrosis: Abnormal enlargement of the kidney and the tube where urine flows, called the ureter.

I

Intraperitoneal: Into the abdomen.

Intraperitoneal port: A device surgically placed under the skin and into the abdomen that allows directed treatment into the abdomen.

Intubation: Process by which a person is placed on a breathing machine.

K

Krukenberg tumor: A cancer that has gone into the ovary from another place, usually starting in the stomach.

L

Laparoscopy: Camera-directed surgery done without creating a large incision in the abdomen.

Laparotomy: Surgery through a large incision in the abdomen.

Lymphatic channels: Vessels through which lymph fluid travels; part of the lymphatic system.

Lymphatic spread: Metastasis of cancer cells through the lymphatic system.

Lymphatic system: A network of lymphatic channels, lymph nodes, and organs, such as the spleen and the tonsils, that forms the major component of the immune system.

M

Menopause: Physical changes marking the end of a woman's fertile years, the most notable change being the cessation of menstrual cycles.

Menstruation: Vaginal bleeding due to endometrial shedding following ovulation when the egg is not fertilized.

Metastases: Tumor that has spread to distant places in the body.

Metastatic: Adjective used to describe a tumor that has spread.

Mitosis: Process of cells dividing.

Mixed mesodermal tumors: Tumors of dual origin with one part consisting of carcinomas and the other part consisting of sarcoma, hence their other designation as a carcinosarcoma.

Moderately differentiated: A pathologist's term to describe cellular changes of a cancer cell; cells that do not resemble their normal appearance but are still recognizable as related to their normal counterparts.

Multicompartmental: Multiple spaces, used to describe a finding

seen in complex cysts on imaging studies, like ultrasounds.

Mutations: Genetic changes in DNA; mutations are not always harmful but sometimes can be associated with cancer development.

Myelodysplastic syndrome: Abnormal development of blood cells that represents a problem in the bone marrow.

N

Nasogastric (NG) tube: A tube placed temporarily through the nose (naso) into the stomach (gastric) to help relieve continuous vomiting caused by a bowel obstruction.

Neoadjuvant treatment: Treatment given before surgery.

O

Omental cake: Tumor involvement of the omentum that results in the formation of a large mass.

Omentum: Fatty apron that drapes from the stomach and colon.

Optimal debulking: Surgical result if residual tumor is less than 1cm in diameter at the end of surgery.

Ovulation: Process of egg release from the ovary.

P

Palliation: To provide relief of pain. Adj.: palliative.

Papilla: Budding formations on structures, seen on ultrasound or other imaging.

Paracentesis: The process of removing ascites.

Patient-controlled analgesia (PCA): A method of providing pain medication through the vein that allows direct control over the amount required to make one comfortable.

Percutaneous endoscopic gastrostomy (PEG): A tube placed by a gastroenterologist that is inserted through your skin (percutaneous) and into your stomach using a flexible tube containing a camera (endoscopic). A hole is made in the stomach (gastrotomy) and the tube is fixed from the stomach and exits the skin. The purpose is to allow continuous drainage of bowel contents in a woman with terminal cancer who has an intractable bowel obstruction.

Perforation: Rupture of the wall of the bowel.

Performance status: A numerical description of how a person is doing in her normal day-to-day life and whether her cancer is impacting her ability to live normally.

Peritoneal carcinomatosis: Involvement of the omentum or bowels with cancer, usually the size of "rice granules" or tumor nodules.

Peritoneal cavity: The abdominal space.

Peritoneal seeding: The process of cancer spreading to involve the peritoneal surface.

Peritoneum: The lining of the peritoneal cavity.

Platinum-resistant: Term used to describe women with recurrent ovarian cancer who relapse less than six months after the end of prior platinum-based treatment.

Platinum-sensitive: Term used to describe women with recurrent ovarian cancer who recurred six months or longer after the end of prior treatment with a platinum agent (e.g., carboplatin).

Pleural effusion: Fluid build-up around the lungs.

Pleurodesis: Process performed to prevent further build-up of fluid around the lung.

Poly-ADP ribose polymerase (PARP) inhibitors: They block proteins involved in the repair of DNA breaks.

Poorly differentiated: A pathologist's term to describe cellular changes of a cancer cell; this describes cells that bear no resemblance to their normal counterparts.

Primary peritoneal cancer: Cancer that arises from the lining of the gut, or the peritoneum. This cancer behaves similarly to ovarian cancer and is treated much in the same way.

Prognosis: An estimate of the outlook following the diagnosis of a disease such as cancer.

Progression-free survival: The time interval between the start of a treatment and when the disease starts to grow once more.

Prophylactic oophorectomy: Removal of a woman's ovaries in an attempt to reduce or remove a risk for ovarian cancer in the future.

Proteinuria: The spilling of protein by the kidneys, which is picked up by a urine evaluation.

Proteomics: The study of protein profiles.

Pulmonary fibrosis: Scarring of the lung tissue, which may or may not be reversible.

R

Regeneration: To grow back.

Renin: A hormone released by the kidney normally that is important in maintaining hydration.

Reservoir: A receptacle that holds fluid.

S

Salpingectomy: Removal of the fallopian tube.

Second-line chemotherapy: Chemotherapy given during recurrence.

Sensory neuropathy: Numbness and tingling, usually involving the hands and feet.

Septations: Thin membranes or walls dividing an area into multiple chambers. Often used to describe complex cysts seen on ultrasound.

Serological relapse: Diagnosis of recurrence solely based on an elevation of a tumor marker without evidence of recurrence by radiology tests.

Sporadic: Isolated; to occur without a pattern.

Suboptimal debulking: Residual disease greater than 1 cm in diameter upon completion of surgery.

Surgical staging: Procedure of determining the extent of cancer present.

T

T-cells: Immune cells that primarily fight viruses. They are being used in clinical trials of immunotherapy for ovarian and other cancers.

Thoracentesis: Procedure of draining a pleural effusion.

Thoracic surgeon: A surgeon who has completed extra training in the surgical management of diseases involving the chest and its organs.

Torsion: Act of twisting or turning in on itself (ovarian torsion, for example).

Total hysterectomy: Surgical excision of the uterus and cervix.

Total parenteral nutrition (TPN): Nutrition that is given by vein.

Treatment-free interval: The time between the end of one chemotherapy regimen and initiation of a subsequent therapy for recurrent disease.

Treatment holiday: A break in treatment that allows the body time to recover from toxicity.

True negative rate: The proportion of patients who have a negative test result and who do not have the disease.

True positive rate: The proportion of patients who have a positive test result and who do have the disease.

Tumor: A mass of cells that grow abnormally.

U

Undifferentiated: A pathologist's term to describe cellular changes of a cancer cell; this describes cells that bear no resemblance at all to normal cells.

Ureter: The anatomical structure that enables us to get rid of urine. It connects the kidney to the bladder.

V

Vaccine: A preparation that is given to induce immunity to a disease or condition.

W

Well-differentiated: A pathologist's term to describe cellular changes of a cancer cell; this describes cells that meet the criteria for cancer but still maintain a resemblance to normal cells.

GLOSSARY

Note: Page numbers followed by *f* and *t* indicate materials in figures and tables respectively.